Self-Assessment Review
Small Animal Imaging

Also available in the Veterinary Self-Assessment Color Review series:

Self-Assessment Review

Small Animal Imaging

John S. Mattoon
DVM, DACVR
Washington State University
College of Veterinary Medicine
Pullman, Washington, USA

Dana A. Neelis
DVM, MS, DACVR
Animal Imaging
Irving, Texas, USA

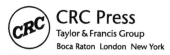

CRC Press
Taylor & Francis Group
Boca Raton London New York

CRC Press is an imprint of the
Taylor & Francis Group, an **informa** business

CRC Press
Taylor & Francis Group
6000 Broken Sound Parkway NW, Suite 300
Boca Raton, FL 33487-2742

© 2018 by Taylor & Francis Group, LLC
CRC Press is an imprint of Taylor & Francis Group, an Informa business

No claim to original U.S. Government works

Printed on acid-free paper

International Standard Book Number-13: 978-1-4822-2520-4 (Paperback)
International Standard Book Number-13: 978-1-138-09149-8 (Hardback)

**Visit the Taylor & Francis Web site at
http://www.taylorandfrancis.com**

**and the CRC Press Web site at
http://www.crcpress.com**

Contents

Preface

This book was conceived as a way of providing students of small animal veterinary medicine a practical 'pocket book' of common diseases that may manifest as abnormalities on a radiographic examination.

The book is in no way intended to be a textbook of radiographic imaging, as there are a number of fine examples already available. By contrast, the book is arranged as a series of case studies through which students may test their diagnostic radiology skills.

The book is divided into three basic sections: thorax, abdomen, and musculoskeletal. The cases are presented as unknowns, with a separate answer section. Each case is presented to the reader as an unknown. A brief signalment and history is given, identical to what was provided when the case was first seen. The radiographic views provided are identified. We ask for radiographic findings followed by a radiographic diagnosis, and in some cases ask if any additional views or studies may be of further value.

Radiographic findings are simply a narrative or list of the abnormalities identified. Sometimes it seems prudent to mention normal findings as well. Incidental abnormal findings on the radiographs are usually noted (e.g. spondylosis in a case of congestive heart failure or pulmonary metastatic disease), although they may not be clinically significant.

The radiographic diagnosis is derived from the radiographic findings. In some cases, a definitive diagnosis can be made with confidence based on the radiographic findings (e.g. a fracture, osteochondritis dissecans, panosteitis). In other cases, a radiographic diagnosis can be made based on the radiographic abnormalities identified in conjunction with the clinical signs and signalment. But in many cases, the radiographic diagnosis is only a concise summary of the findings, which then must be followed by a short list of differential diagnoses. It is in these instances that further imaging procedures, blood work, cytology, biopsy, etc. may be necessary to reach a final diagnosis.

As students of diagnostic imaging, it is vital to do your best to identify radiographic abnormalities (findings) without jumping ahead to the radiographic diagnoses. This is admittedly easier said than done at the beginning, but with practice it can become second nature.

In the answer section, we provide our radiographic findings in a narrative form, using radiology terminology along the way. Please appreciate that this is simply our style of reporting. We do not expect your interpretations to match ours word for word.

Our radiographic diagnoses should be self-explanatory, made based on our abnormal findings. Following our radiographic diagnosis, there may be additional studies to be considered. We have done our best to explain the value of additional studies. In some cases, we provide ultrasound, computed tomography, or magnetic resonance imaging examinations to illustrate how these studies contributed to the case.

For many of the cases presented, a final diagnosis is listed. This is the true diagnosis, based on laboratory work, pathology reports (biopsies, necropsies), etc. As is often the case, the radiographic diagnosis may or may not be the final (true) diagnosis. Frustrating at times, but a real life scenario nonetheless.

Finally, we often offer our thoughts about a case in the comments section.

In the end, the format of the book is a 'written form' of our thought processes as we work through cases every day on the clinic floor. We hope it is helpful, but if not, perhaps it will inspire an alternative approach.

We hope veterinary students find this book valuable when used as intended. We envision it will be passed along from class to class as students progress to higher levels of diagnostic skills during their academic and professional careers.

Have fun!

John S. Mattoon
Dana A. Neelis

Acknowledgments

We wish to express our sincere thanks to the many good people at CRC Press who have lent their considerable expertise and unprecedented patience during the preparation of this book. Jill Northcott, Alice Oven, Paul Bennett, and Peter Beynon, your efforts will always be remembered.

We also offer a huge thank you to Amanda Crabtree, DVM, MS, Diplomate ACVR. Dr. Crabtree was responsible for collecting and cataloging many of the initial images at the inception of this text many years ago.

Broad Classification of Cases

Abdominal masses
2.3, 2.11, 2.15, 2.16, 2.19, 2.20, 2.22, 2.23, 2.31, 2.33, 2.37

Biliary tract
2.24, 2.29, 2.41

Congenital disorders
1.2, 1.14, 1.21, 1.25, 1.26, 1.43

Diaphragmatic disorders
1.15, 1.17, 1.41

Esophageal disorders
1.7, 1.29, 1.42, 1.43, 1.50

Female genital tract
2.2, 2.8, 2.17

Foreign bodies
1.28, 1.42, 2.4, 2.12, 2.25, 2.30, 2.32, 2.33, 2.36, 3.47

Fractures
3.5, 3.9, 3.12, 3.17, 3.20, 3.21, 3.27, 3.31, 3.34, 3.37, 3.42, 3.49, 3.52, 3.56, 3.58

Gastric disease
2.7, 2.14, 2.39

Heart disease
1.2, 1.3, 1.10, 1.12, 1.13, 1.18, 1.21, 1.23, 1.25, 1.26, 1.27, 1.30

Hernias
1.15, 1.17, 1.41, 2.35

Infective disease
1.11, 1.22, 1.33, 1.38, 3.2, 3.36, 3.39

Intestinal disorders
2.1, 2.4, 2.6, 2.21, 2.25, 2.28, 2.30, 2.32, 2.35, 2.36, 2.37

Joint disease
3.3, 3.4, 3.6, 3.7, 3.13, 3.18, 3.22, 3.23, 3.24, 3.26, 3.29, 3.30, 3.32, 3.33, 3.40, 3.41, 3.43, 3.51, 3.54, 3.55

Ligament and tendon disorders
3.7, 3.24, 3.32, 3.45

Lymphadenopathy
1.35, 1.37, 2.16

Mediastinal disease
1.29, 1.46, 1.48, 1.50

Metabolic bone disease
3.54, 3.57

Mineralization
1.20, 2.13, 2.24, 3.1

Neoplasia, thoracic
1.4, 1.16, 1.18, 1.30, 1.34, 1.35, 1.36, 1.48, 1.49

Neoplasia, abdominal
2.3, 2.6, 2.16, 2.22, 2.23, 2.27, 2.31, 2.32, 2.38, 2.39

Neoplasia, musculoskeletal
3.8, 3.10, 3.11, 3.15, 3.20, 3.25, 3.44, 3.46, 3.59

Normal Dog and Cat Anatomy

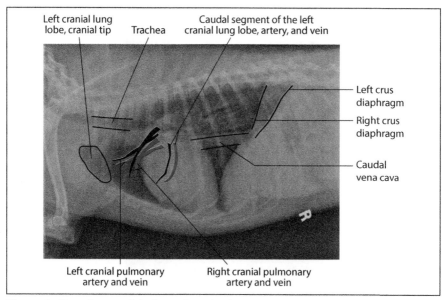

Left cranial lung lobe, cranial tip

Trachea

Caudal segment of the left cranial lung lobe, artery, and vein

Left crus diaphragm

Right crus diaphragm

Caudal vena cava

Left cranial pulmonary artery and vein

Right cranial pulmonary artery and vein

Figure A Dog thorax right lateral projection.

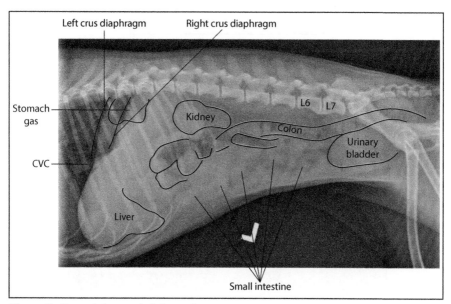

Left crus diaphragm

Right crus diaphragm

Stomach gas

CVC

Kidney

L6 L7

Colon

Urinary bladder

Liver

Small intestine

Figure B Dog abdomen left lateral projection.

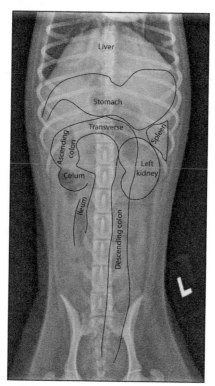

Figure C Dog abdomen ventrodorsal projection.

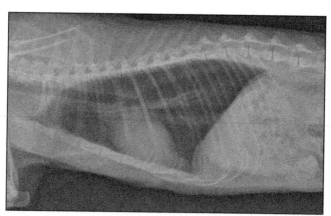

Figure D Cat thorax right lateral projection.

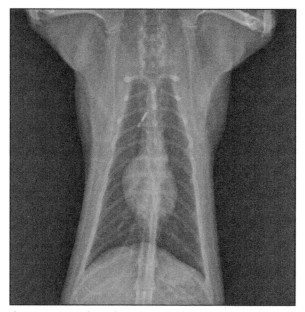

Figure E Cat thorax ventrodorsal projection.

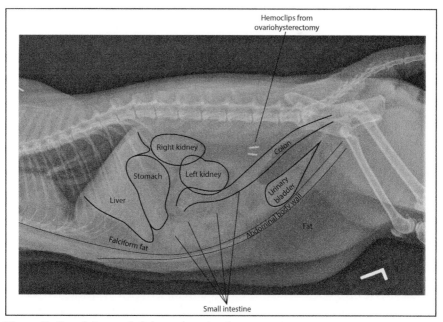

Figure F Cat abdomen left lateral projection.

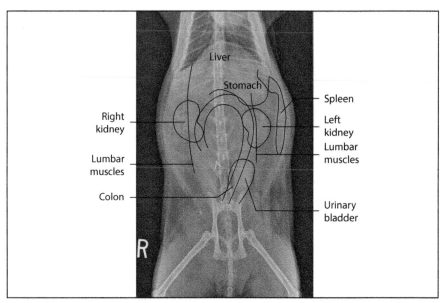

Figure G Cat abdomen ventrodorsal projection.

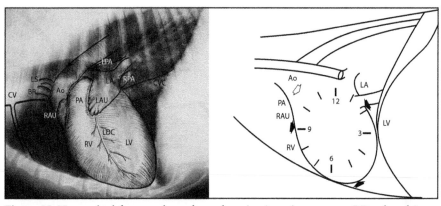

Figure H Heart clockface analogy, lateral projection. Ao = aorta; BR = brachioce-phalic artery; CV = cranial vena cava; LPA = left pulmonary artery; LS = left sub-clavian artery; LAU = left auricle; LA = left atrium; LV = left ventricle; RV = right ventricle; PA = pulmonary artery; CVC = caudal vena cava; RAU = right auricle; RPA = right pulmonary artery.

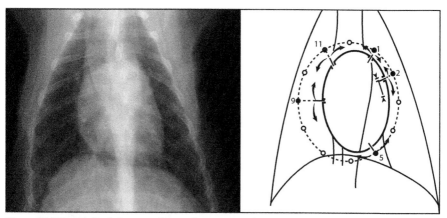

Figure I Heart clockface analogy, dorsoventral projection. 11-1 o'clock position = location of the aortic arch; 1-2 o'clock position = location of the main pulmonary artery; 2-3 o'clock position = area of the left auricle, which will protrude in cases of left atrial enlargement; between 3 and 6 o'clock = left ventricle, including the apex of the heart; between 6 and 9 o'clock = right ventricle; 9 to 11 o'clock = right atrium.

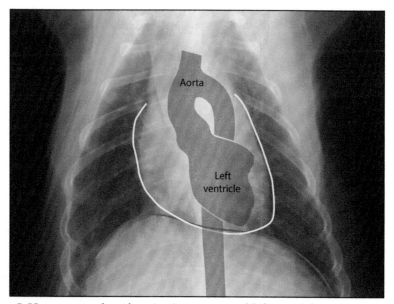

Figure J Heart ventrodorsal projection; aorta and left ventricle.

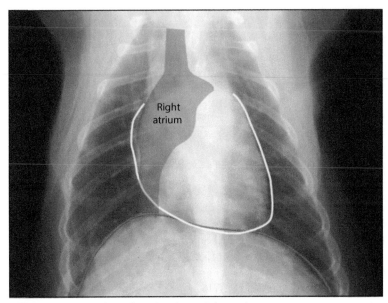

Figure K Heart ventrodorsal projection; right atrium.

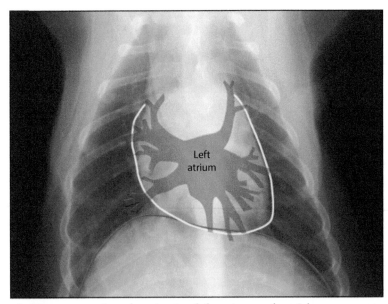

Figure L Heart ventrodorsal projection left atrium and auricle.

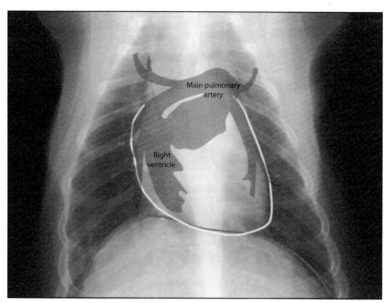

Figure M Heart ventrodorsal projection; right ventricle and main pulmonary artery.

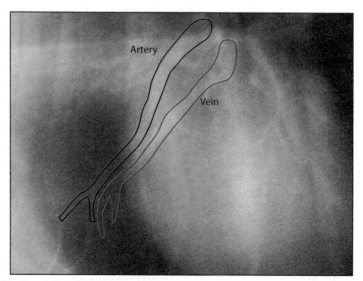

Figure N Cranial pulmonary vessels.

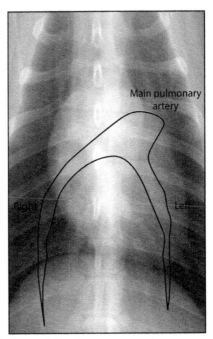

Figure O Right and left caudal pulmonary arteries.

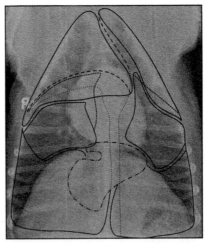

Figure P Surfaces of the lungs. The seven lung lobes of the dog are outlined on the dorsoventral view. These include the right cranial, middle and caudal lobes; the left cranial (cranial and caudal segments) and caudal lobes; and the accessory lung lobe located centrally and caudal to the heart.

CASE 1.1 A 7-year-old neutered male Labrador Retriever who was hit by a car. You obtain these thoracic radiographs: **Figs. 1.1a, b**, left and right lateral projections, respectively; **Figs. 1.1c, d**, ventrodorsal and dorsoventral projections, respectively.

1 What are your radiographic findings?
2 What is your radiographic diagnosis?

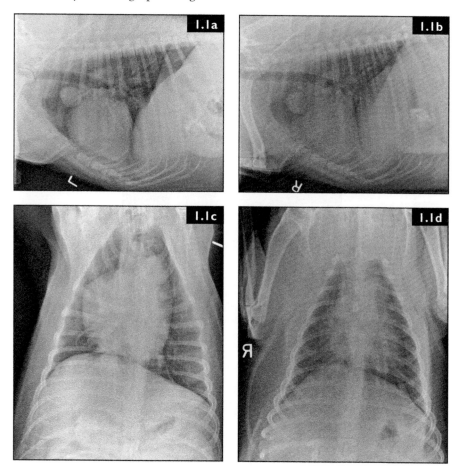

CASE 1.2 A 4-month-old female domestic shorthair cat with shallow breathing and a grade III/VI continuous murmur at the left cranial base. You obtain these thoracic radiographs: **Fig. 1.2a**, right lateral projection; **Fig. 1.2b**, dorsoventral projection.

1 What are your radiographic findings?
2 What is your radiographic diagnosis?
3 Is additional imaging needed?

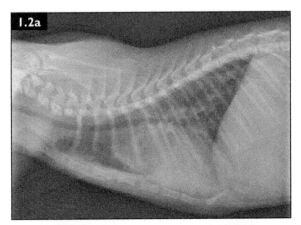

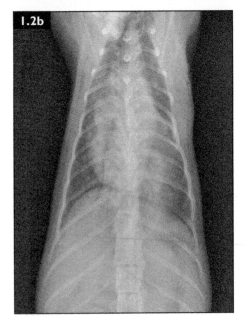

CASE 1.3 An 8-year-old male German Shepherd Dog with lethargy and muffled heart sounds. No heart murmur ausculted. You obtain these thoracic radiographs: **Fig. 1.3a**, left lateral projection; **Fig. 1.3b**, dorsoventral projection.

1 What are your radiographic findings?
2 What is your radiographic diagnosis?
3 Is additional imaging needed?

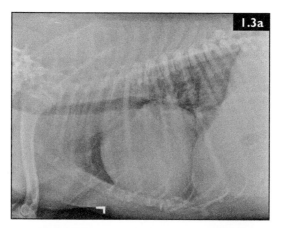

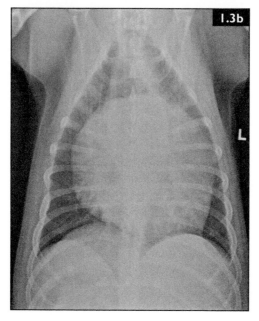

CASE 1.4 A 13-year-old spayed female mixed breed dog with a history of polyuria and polydipsia and abdominal distension. You obtain these thoracic radiographs: **Fig. 1.4a**, left lateral projection; **Fig. 1.4b**, dorsoventral projection.

1 What are your radiographic findings?
2 What is your radiographic diagnosis?
3 Are any additional radiographs needed?

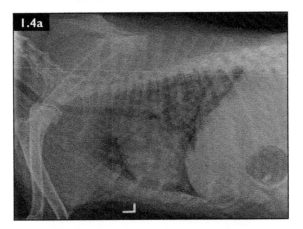

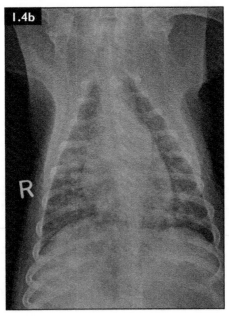

CASE 1.5 An 8-year-old spayed female English Mastiff with a 2-week history of labored breathing, anorexia, and weight loss. You obtain these thoracic radiographs: **Fig. 1.5a**, right lateral projection; **Fig. 1.5b**, dorsoventral projection.

1 What are your radiographic findings?
2 What is your radiographic diagnosis?

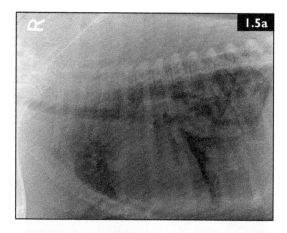

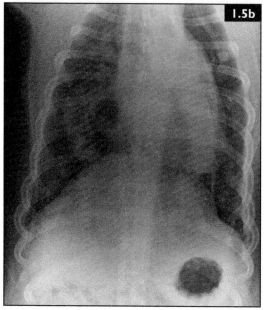

CASE 1.6 A 10-week-old male Beagle with abnormal mentation, tachypnea, and ptyalism. On physical examination, a hemorrhagic and erythematous lesion is found in the oral cavity. You obtain these thoracic radiographs: **Figs. 1.6a, b,** left lateral and right lateral projections, respectively; **1.6c,** dorsoventral projection.

1 What are your radiographic findings?
2 What is your radiographic diagnosis?
3 Are any additional radiographic views needed?

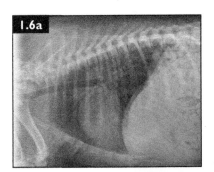
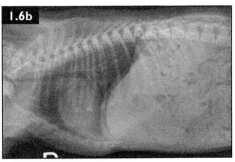
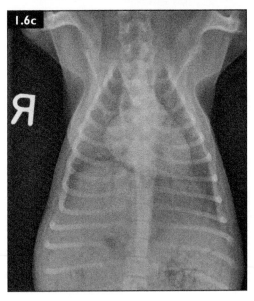

CASE 1.7 A 9-year-old spayed female Vizla with a 3-week history of stumbling and weakness following exercise and regurgitation following eating. You obtain these thoracic radiographs: **Figs. 1.7a, b,** left and right lateral projections, respectively; **Fig. 1.7c,** dorsoventral projection.

1 What are your radiographic findings?
2 What is your radiographic diagnosis?

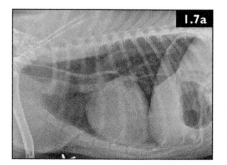
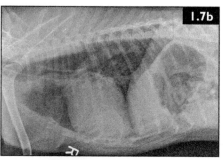
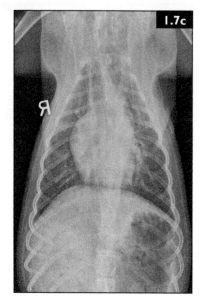

CASE 1.8 A 12-year-old neutered male Jack Russell Terrier with a productive cough. You obtain these thoracic radiographs: **Figs. 1.8a, b,** left and right lateral projections, respectively; **Fig. 1.8c,** ventrodorsal projection.

1 What are your radiographic findings?
2 What is your radiographic diagnosis?

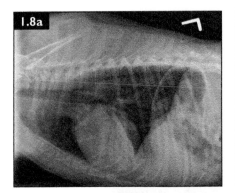

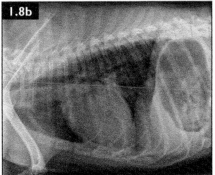

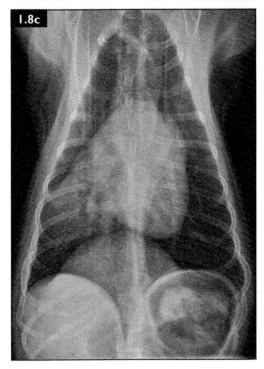

CASE 1.9 A 10-year-old neutered male Golden Retriever with labored breathing and exercise intolerance. You obtain these throacic radiographs: **Fig. 1.9a**, left lateral projection; **Fig. 1.9b**, dorsoventral projection.

1 What are your radiographic findings?
2 What is your radiographic diagnosis?
3 Are additional radiographic projections needed?

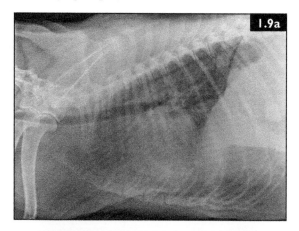

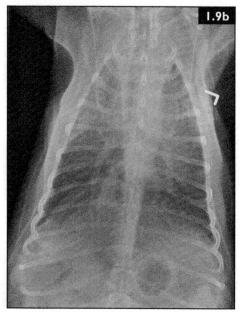

CASE 1.10 A 3-year-old neutered male domestic shorthair cat with acute hindlimb paralysis and tachycardia. You obtain these thoracic radiographs: **Fig. 1.10a**, left lateral projection; **Fig. 1.10b**, dorsoventral projection.

1 What are your radiographic findings?
2 What is your radiographic diagnosis?
3 Is additional imaging needed?

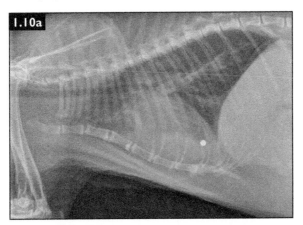

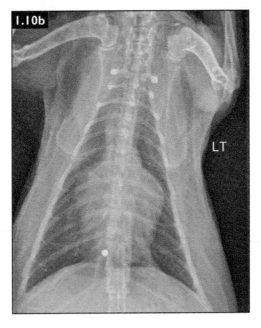

CASE 1.11 A 4-year-old female German Shorthair Pointer with a 1-week history of a cough, dyspnea, and lethargy. You obtain these thoracic radiographs: **Figs. 1.11a, b,** left and right lateral projections, respectively; **Fig. 1.11c,** ventrodorsal projection.

1 What are your radiographic findings?
2 What is your radiographic diagnosis?

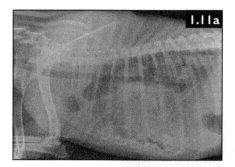
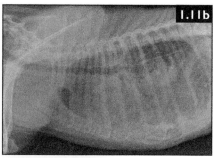
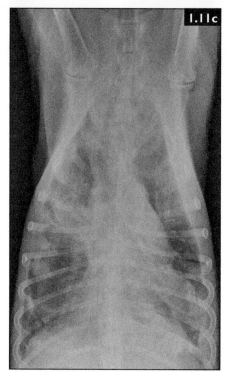

CASE 1.12 A 9-year-old spayed female cat with a cough and lethargy. Crackles and wheezes were auscultated on physical examination. You obtain these thoracic radiographs: **Fig. 1.12a**, right lateral projection; **1.12b**, dorsoventral projection.

1 What are your radiographic findings?
2 What is your radiographic diagnosis?
3 Is further imaging needed?

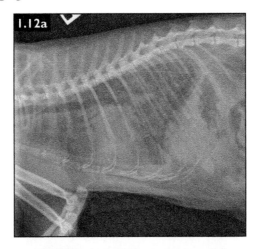

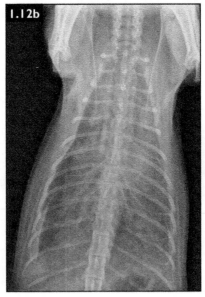

CASE 1.13 A 3-month-old male Newfoundland with episodes of weakness with cyanosis and an occasional, dry cough. On auscultation, a grade V/VI holosystolic basilar murmur was identified. You obtain these thoracic radiographs: **Fig. 1.13a**, right lateral projection; **1.13b**, dorsoventral projection.

1 What are your radiographic findings?
2 What is your radiographic diagnosis?
3 Is further imaging needed?

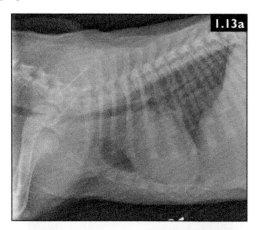

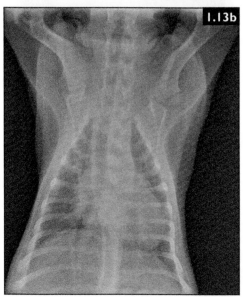

CASE 1.14 A 5-month-old female Shetland Sheepdog with exercise intolerance and shortness of breath. You obtain these thoracic radiographs: **Figs. 1.14a, b,** left and right lateral projections, respectively; **Fig. 1.14c,** dorsoventral projection.

1 What are your radiographic findings?
2 What is your radiographic diagnosis?

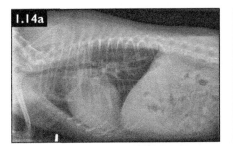

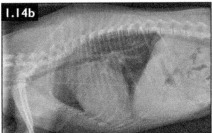

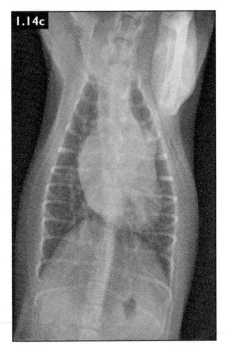

CASE 1.15 A 2-year-old neutered male mixed breed canine with intermittent vomiting, which has recently increased to three times daily, and muffled heart sounds. You obtain these thoracic radiographs: **Fig. 1.15a**, left lateral projection; **Fig. 1.15b**, dorsoventral projection.

1 What are your radiographic findings?
2 What is your radiographic diagnosis?
3 Is additional imaging needed?

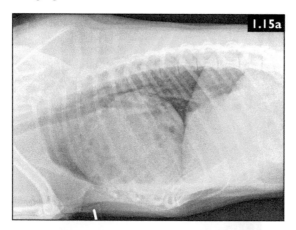

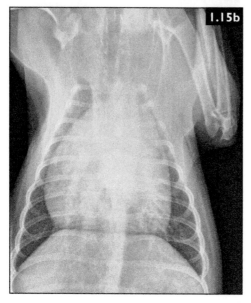

CASE 1.16 A 12-year-old neutered male domestic shorthair cat with a 3-week history of swelling of the left rear foot and anorexia. You obtain these thoracic radiographs: **Fig. 1.16a**, left lateral projection; **Fig. 1.16b**, dorsoventral projection.

1 What are your radiographic findings?
2 What is your radiographic diagnosis?
3 Are additional radiographs needed?

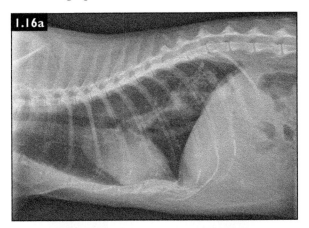

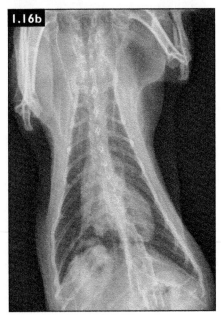

CASE 1.17 A 3-year-old neutered male Shih Tzu with a 5-day history of tachypnea, back pain, and anorexia. You obtain these thoracic radiographs: **Figs. 1.17a, b,** left and right lateral projections, respectively; **Fig. 1.17c,** dorsoventral projection.

1 What are your radiographic findings?
2 What is your radiographic diagnosis?
3 Is additional imaging needed?

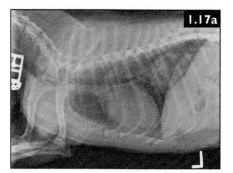

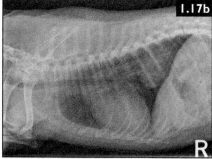

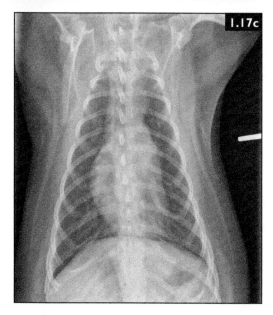

CASE 1.18 A 10-year-old spayed female Cocker Spaniel with a history of having dyspneic episodes when stressed. You obtain these thoracic radiographs: **Figs. 1.18a,b**, left and right lateral projections, respectively; **Fig. 1.18c**, ventrodorsal projection.

1 What are your radiographic findings?
2 What is your radiographic diagnosis?

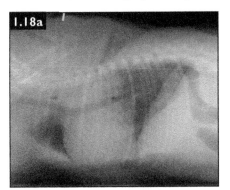
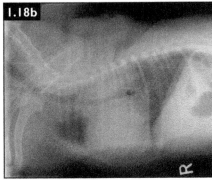
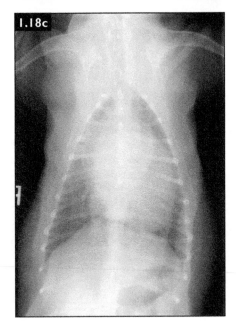

CASE 1.19 A 13-year-old neutered male Siamese with a chronic cough, lethargy, and tachypnea. You obtain these thoracic radiographs: **Fig. 1.19a**, left lateral projection; **Figs. 1.19b, c**, ventrodorsal and dorsoventral projections, respectively.

1 What are your radiographic findings?
2 What is your radiographic diagnosis?

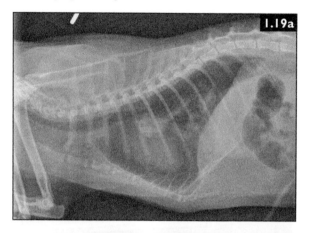

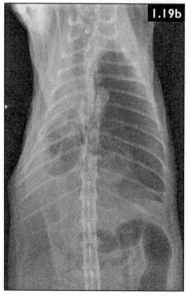 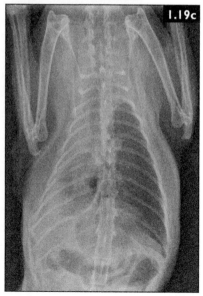

CASE 1.20 A 10-year-old spayed female Rottweiler with a chronic cough. You obtain these thoracic radiographs: **Fig. 1.20a**, left lateral projection; **Fig. 1.20b**, dorsoventral projection.

1 What are your radiographic findings?
2 What is your radiographic diagnosis?

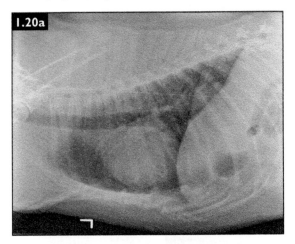

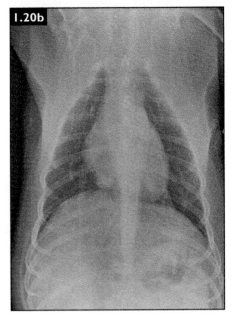

CASE 1.21 A 2-month-old female Boxer with two episodes of collapse. You obtain these thoracic radiographs: **Fig. 1.21a**, right lateral projection; **Fig. 1.21b**, dorsoventral projection.

1 What are your radiographic findings?
2 What is your radiographic diagnosis?
3 Is additional imaging needed?

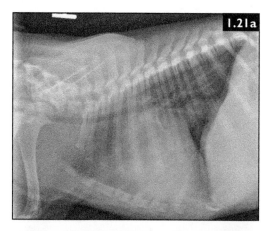

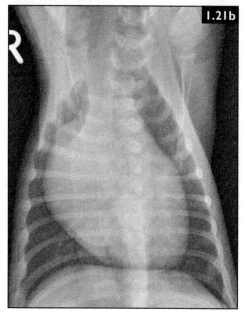

CASE **1.22** A 4-year-old spayed female Labrador Retriever with chronic coughing. You obtain these thoracic radiographs: **Figs. 1.22a, b,** left and right lateral projections, respectively; **Fig. 1.22c,** dorsoventral projection.

1 What are your radiographic findings?
2 What is your radiographic diagnosis?

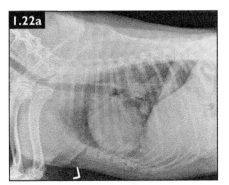

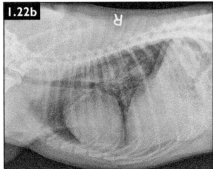

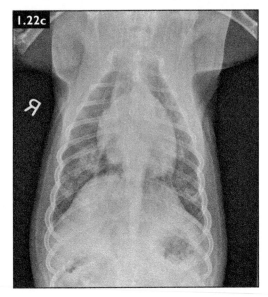

CASE 1.23 A 6-year-old neutered male Doberman Pinscher with a productive cough and distended abdomen. You obtain these thoracic radiographs: **Fig. 1.23a**, left lateral projection; **Figs. 1.23b, c,** ventrodorsal and dorsoventral projections, respectively.

1 What are your radiographic findings?
2 What is your radiographic diagnosis?

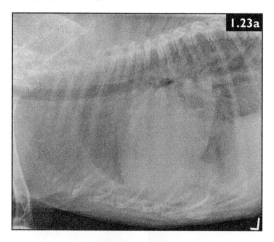

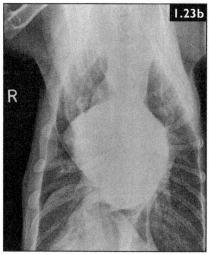

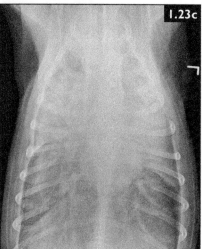

CASE 1.24 A 7-year-old female Brittany with anorexia and dyspnea. You obtain these thoracic radiographs: **Fig. 1.24a**, right lateral projection; **Fig. 1.24b**, ventrodorsal projection; **Fig. 1.24c**, close up lateral view of the lung pattern.

1 What are your radiographic findings?
2 What is your radiographic diagnosis?

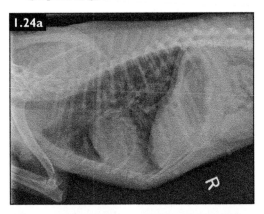

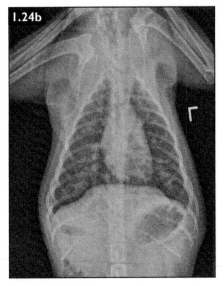

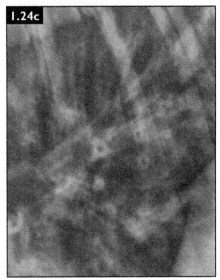

CASE 1.25 A 7-month-old male German Shepherd Dog with a history of lethargy and a grade V/VI left basilar systolic murmur. You obtain these thoracic radiographs: **Figs. 1.25a, b,** left and right lateral projections, respectively; **Fig. 1.25c,** dorsoventral projection.

1 What are your radiographic findings?
2 What is your radiographic diagnosis?
3 Is additional imaging needed?

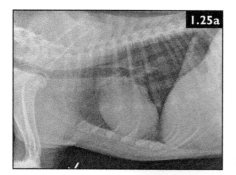
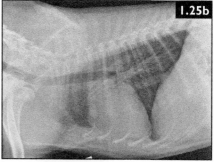
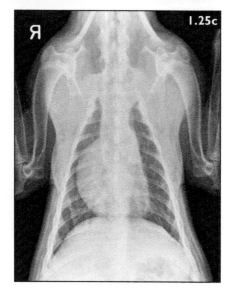

CASE 1.26 A 7-week-old female domestic shorthair cat with a grade VI/VI systolic heart murmur heard best at the right cranial border. You obtain these thoracic radiographs: **Fig. 1.26a**, left lateral projection; **Fig. 1.26b**, dorsoventral projection.

1 What are your radiographic findings?
2 What is your radiographic diagnosis?
3 Is additional imaging needed?

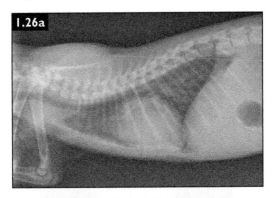

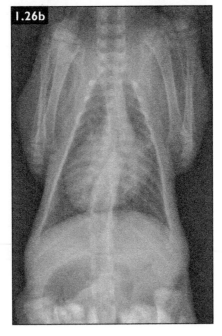

CASE 1.27 An 8-year-old spayed female Shetland Sheepdog with a history of vestibular neurologic signs, tetraparesis, decreased proprioception, and a decreased menace response. These thoracic radiographs are obtained prior to magnetic resonance imaging examination: **Fig. 1.27a**, right lateral projection; **Fig. 1.27b**, ventrodorsal projection.

1 What are your radiographic findings?
2 What is your radiographic diagnosis?

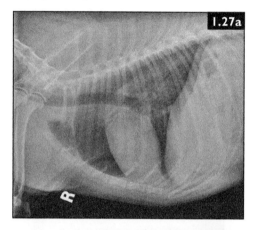

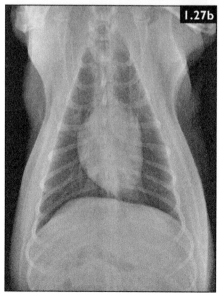

CASE 1.28 A 2-year-old neutered male cat with an acute onset of dyspnea. You obtain these thoracic radiographs: **Figs. 1.28a, b,** left and right lateral projections, respectively; **Fig. 1.28c,** ventrodorsal projection.

1 What are your radiographic findings?
2 What is your radiographic diagnosis?

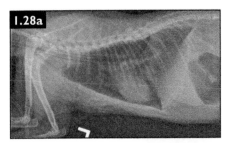

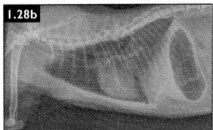

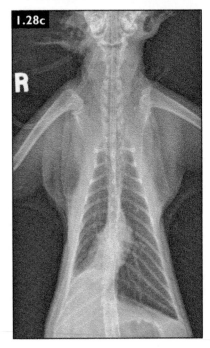

CASE 1.29 A 7-year-old spayed female mixed breed dog with a history of regurgitation. You obtain these thoracic radiographs: **Fig. 1.29a**, left lateral projection; **Fig. 1.29b**, ventrodorsal projection.

1 What are your radiographic findings?
2 What is your radiographic diagnosis?

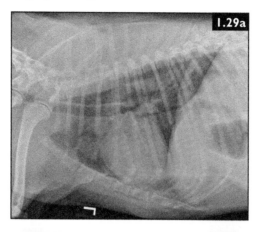

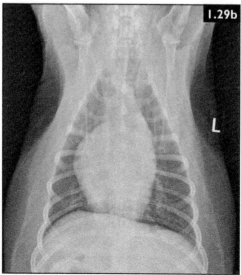

CASE 1.30 An 11-year-old spayed female Labrador cross with a heart murmur. You obtain these thoracic radiographs: **Fig. 1.30a**, left lateral projection; **Fig. 1.30b**, ventrodorsal projection.

1 What are your radiographic findings?
2 What is your radiographic diagnosis?
3 Is additional imaging needed?

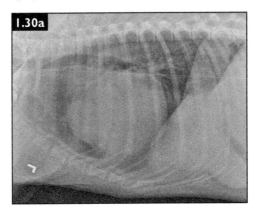

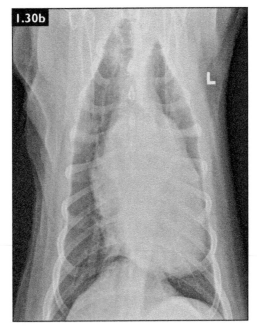

CASE 1.31 A 10-year-old spayed female Lhasa Apso dog with a cough and heart murmur. You obtain these thoracic radiographs: **Fig. 1.31a**, left lateral projection; **Fig. 1.31b**, dorsoventral projection.

1   What are your radiographic findings?
2   What is your radiographic diagnosis?
3   Is additional imaging needed?

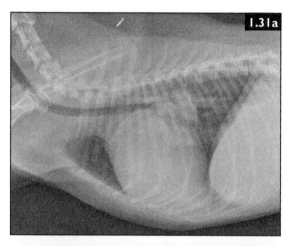

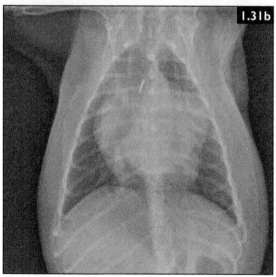

CASE 1.32 A 2-year-old spayed female Abyssinian cat with dyspnea. You obtain these thoracic radiographs: **Fig. 1.32a**, left lateral projection; **Fig. 1.32b**, dorsoventral projection.

1 What are your radiographic findings?
2 What is your radiographic diagnosis?

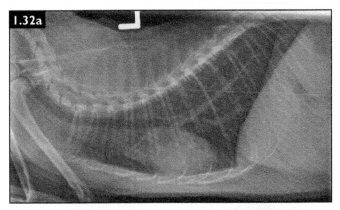

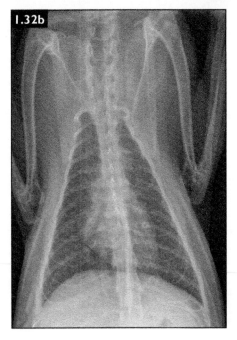

CASE 1.33 A 7-year-old neutered male domestic shorthair cat with dyspnea and coughing. You obtain these thoracic radiographs: **Figs. 1.33a, b,** left and right lateral projections, respectively; **Fig. 1.33c,** dorsoventral projection.

1 What are your radiographic findings?
2 What is your radiographic diagnosis?

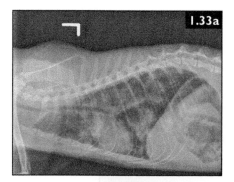
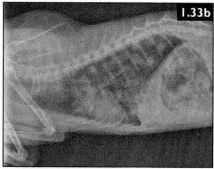
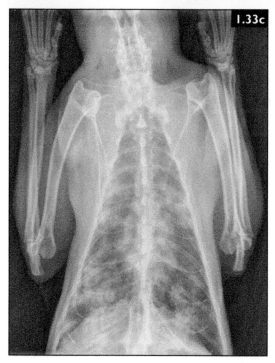

CASE 1.34 A 7-year-old spayed female mixed breed canine with anorexia, lethargy, weight loss, tachypnea, and cranial abdominal organomegaly. You obtain these thoracic radiographs: **Fig. 1.34a**, right lateral projection; **Fig. 1.34b**, dorsoventral projection.

1 What are your radiographic findings?
2 What is your radiographic diagnosis?

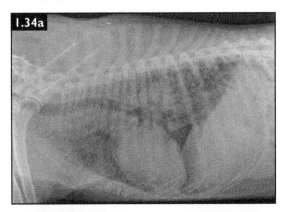

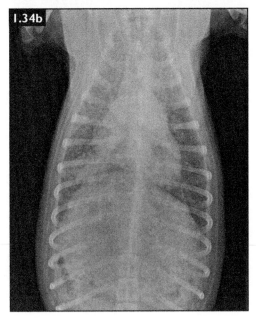

CASE 1.35 A 10-year-old male neutered Greyhound with a grade I/VI left basilar systolic heart murmur and a previous diagnosis of pleural and pericardial effusion. You obtain these thoracic radiographs: **Fig. 1.35a,** right lateral projection; **Fig. 1.35b,** ventrodorsal projection.

1 What are your radiographic findings?
2 What is your radiographic diagnosis?

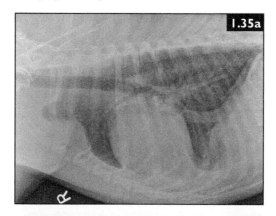

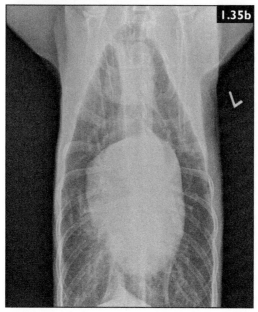

CASE 1.36 A 4-year-old female Mastiff with a prior diagnosis of osteosarcoma of the left hindlimb, which was amputated 1 year ago. You obtain these thoracic radiographs: **Fig. 1.36a**, right lateral projection; **Fig. 1.36b**, dorsoventral projection.

1 What are your radiographic findings?
2 What is your radiographic diagnosis?

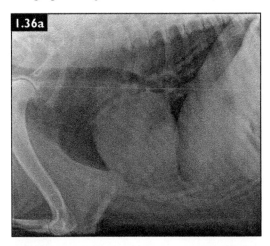

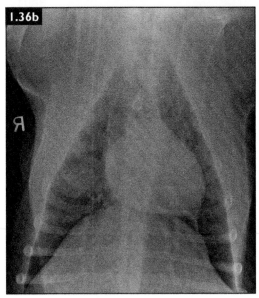

CASE 1.37 A 5-year-old male neutered Shiz Tzu with a cough. You obtain these thoracic radiographs: **Fig. 1.37a**, right lateral projection; **Fig. 1.37b**, ventrodorsal projection.

1 What are your radiographic findings?
2 What is your radiographic diagnosis?

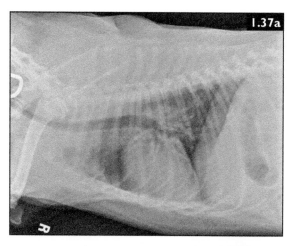

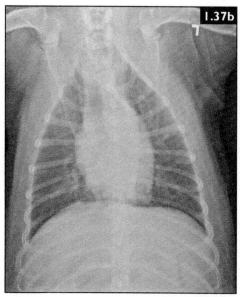

CASE 1.38 A 1-year-old spayed female domestic shorthair cat with severe respiratory distress. You obtain these thoracic radiographs: **Fig. 1.38a**, left lateral projection; **Fig. 1.38b**, ventrodorsal projection.

1 What are your radiographic findings?
2 What is your radiographic diagnosis?

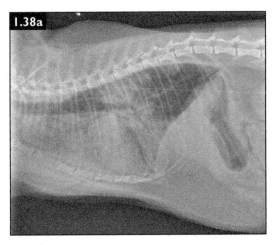

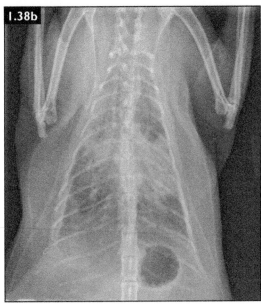

CASE 1.39 A 12-year-old spayed female Golden Retriever with a history of anorexia, vomiting, and increased respiratory rate. You obtain these thoracic radiographs: **Fig. 1.39a**, left lateral projection; **Fig. 1.39b**, ventrodorsal projection.

1 What are your radiographic findings?
2 What is your radiographic diagnosis?

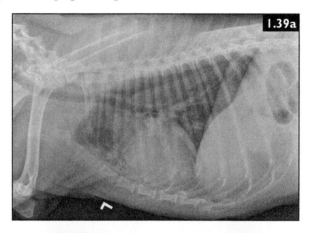

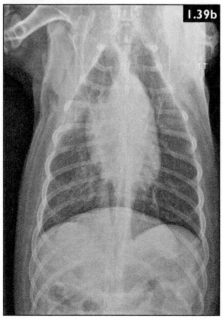

CASE 1.40 A 3-year-old male neutered Australian Cattle Dog with left nasal discharge and epistaxis. You obtain these thoracic radiographs: **Figs. 1.40a, b,** left and right lateral projections, respectively; **Fig. 1.40c,** dorsoventral projection.

1 What are your radiographic findings?
2 What is your radiographic diagnosis?

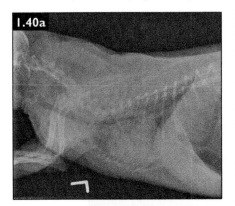

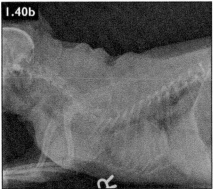

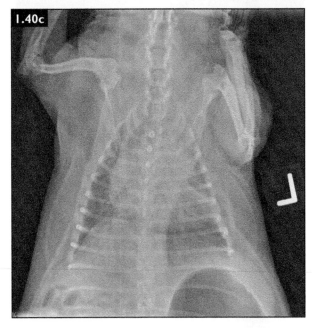

CASE 1.41 A 7-month-old male Labrador Retriever puppy with acute respiratory distress after a hike. You obtain these thoracic radiographs: **Fig. 1.41a**, right lateral projection; **Fig. 1.41b**, dorsoventral projection.

1 What are your radiographic findings?
2 What is your radiographic diagnosis?
3 Is additional imaging needed?

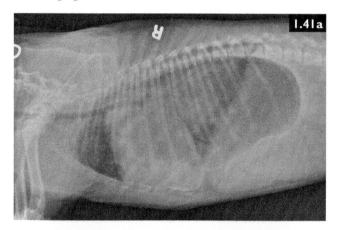

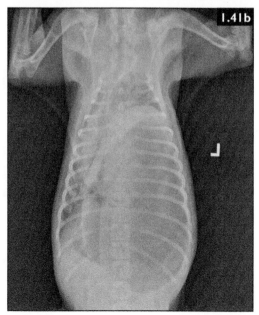

41

CASE 1.42 A 4-year-old spayed female Labrador Retriever with a history of retching and restlessness that started this afternoon. You obtain these thoracic radiographs: **Fig. 1.42a**, left lateral projection; **Fig. 1.42b**, ventrodorsal projection.

1 What are your radiographic findings?
2 What is your radiographic diagnosis?
3 Is additional imaging needed?

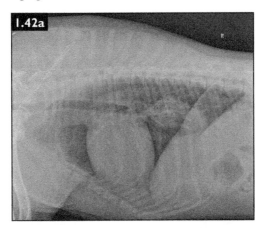

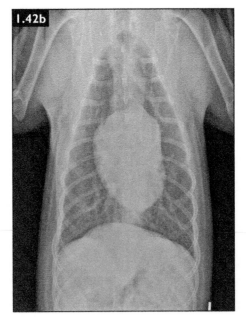

CASE 1.43 A 3-month-old female Boston Terrier with a history of regurgitation. You obtain these thoracic radiographs: Fig. 1.43a, right lateral projection; Fig. 1.43b, ventrodorsal projection.

1 What are your radiographic findings?
2 What is your radiographic diagnosis?
3 Is additional imaging needed?

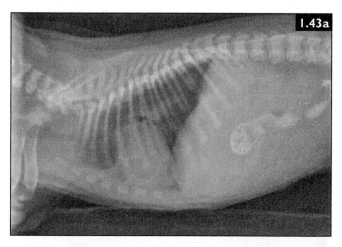

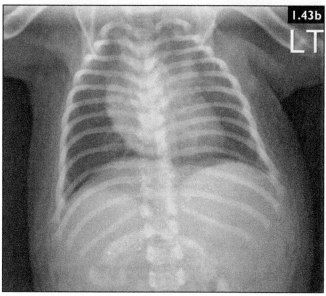

CASE 1.44 A 7-month-old male mixed breed dog who was recently hit by a car and is now dyspneic. You obtain these thoracic radiographs: **Fig. 1.44a**, left lateral projection; **Fig. 1.44b**, dorsoventral projection.

1 What are your radiographic findings?
2 What is your radiographic diagnosis?

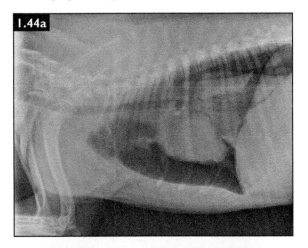

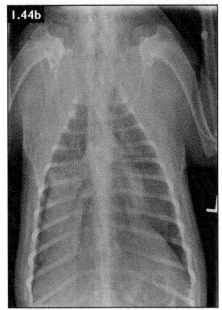

CASE 1.45 A 13-year-old male neutered American Cocker Spaniel who presented for a dental examination and a heart murmur was ausculted. You obtain these thoracic radiographs: **Fig. 1.45a**, left lateral projection; **Fig. 1.45b**, ventrodorsal projection.

1 What are your radiographic findings?
2 What is your radiographic diagnosis?

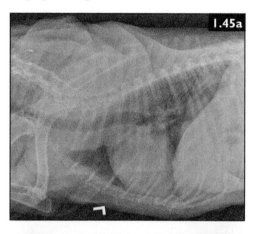

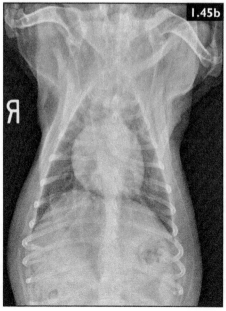

CASE 1.46 A 4-year-old male neutered Chihuahua with tachypnea following an attack by a larger dog. You obtain these thoracic radiographs: **Fig. 1.46a**, right lateral projection; **Fig. 1.46b**, ventrodorsal projection.

1 What are your radiographic findings?
2 What is your radiographic diagnosis?

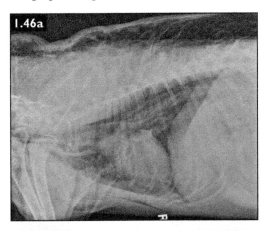

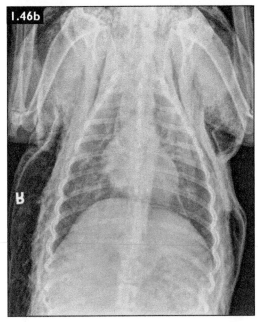

CASE 1.47 A 6-year-old spayed female Bassett Hound with a history of tachypnea. You obtain these thoracic radiographs: **Fig. 1.47a**, left lateral projection; **Fig. 1.47b**, dorsoventral projection.

1 What are your radiographic findings?
2 What is your radiographic diagnosis?

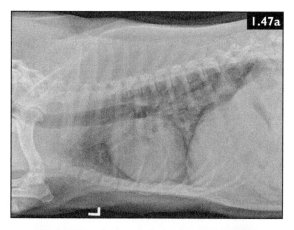

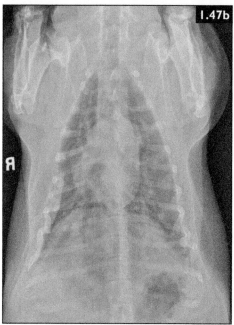

CASE 1.48 A 9-year-old spayed female Labrador Retriever with occasional dyspnea and a cough. You obtain these thoracic radiographs: Fig. 1.48a, right lateral projection; Fig. 1.48b, dorsoventral projection.

1 What are your radiographic findings?
2 What is your radiographic diagnosis?
3 Is additional imaging needed?

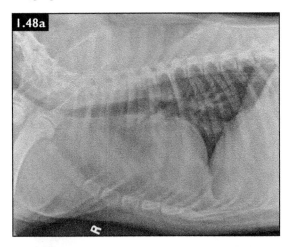

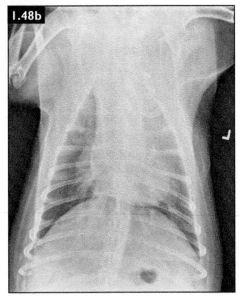

CASE 1.49 A 12-year-old male castrated Maltese with a history of a cough. You obtain these thoracic radiographs: **Fig. 1.49a**, left lateral projection; **Fig. 1.49b**, ventrodorsal projection.

1 What are your radiographic findings?
2 What is your radiographic diagnosis?

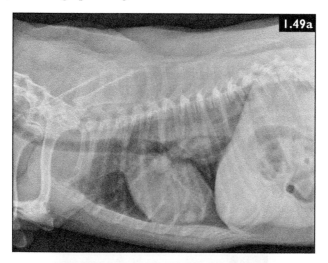

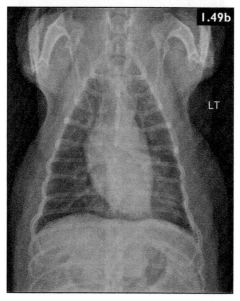

CASE 1.50 A 5-year-old neutered male mixed breed dog with coughing and regurgitation. You obtain these thoracic radiographs: **Fig. 1.50a**, right lateral projection; **Fig. 1.50b**, ventrodorsal projection.

1 What are your radiographic findings?
2 What is your radiographic diagnosis?
3 Is additional imaging needed?

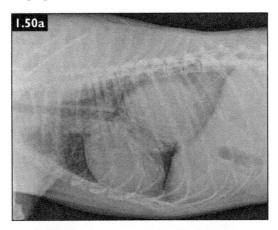

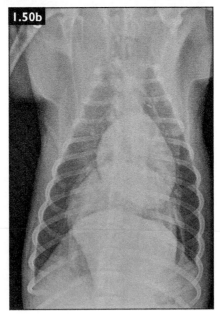

CASE 1.1

1 What are your radiographic findings? An approximately 4 cm mass (nodule) is present in the left cranial lung lobe, located near the midline. No other abnormalities are identified.

2 What is your radiographic diagnosis? Solitary left cranial lung lobe mass. Differential diagnosis: given the clinical history, a solitary hematoma is considered, although pulmonary contusion is usually more diffuse and less structured. The mass may be a solitary pulmonary neoplasm (e.g. primary lung tumor), a cyst, granulomas, or a focus of infection.

Note how this large mass is difficult to identify on the dorsoventral view, and even more hidden on the ventrodorsal projection. In this case, the two lateral views show a nearly identical appearance of the mass.

Final diagnosis: A cranial left lobectomy was performed. The mass was diagnosed as a *Paragonimus* cyst.

CASE 1.2

1 What are your radiographic findings? The cardiac silhouette is markedly enlarged, occupying the majority of the thorax. It is too tall and too wide. There is dorsal displacement of the trachea, nearly parallel to the spine on the lateral view. Note how long and how wide the heart appears on the dorsoventral view and the apex is rounded. On the lateral view the cardiac silhouette has assumed a more horizontal position within the thorax. The severe cardiac enlargement has resulted in increased cardiophrenic and cardiosternal contact. There is an abnormal leftward bulge of the proximal portion of the descending aorta on the dorsoventral view. The pulmonary blood vessels are very enlarged. The dorsoventral view shows enlargement of the right and left caudal lobar artery and vein pairs. The caudal pulmonary blood vessels margins are partially obscured, making them more difficult to see than the cranial pair. This is due to a mild interstitial pulmonary infiltrate present in the caudal lung lobes; the cranial lobes do not show this infiltrate. There is also partially silhouetting with the apical portion of the heart margins because of this interstitial infiltrate.

2 What is your radiographic diagnosis? Severe cardiac enlargement with pulmonary overcirculation and heart failure. The most likely diagnosis is the congenital heart defect, left-to-right patent ductus arteriosus (PDA). This radiographic diagnosis can be made with confidence. Key findings for a diagnosis of PDA are overcirculation (arteries and veins are enlarged), the identified 'ductus bump' on the descending aorta, and the auscultated continuous heart murmur. The interstitial pattern represents pulmonary edema consistent with left-sided congestive heart failure.

3 Is additional imaging needed? Echocardiography should be preformed to confirm the diagnosis, obtain baseline data to assess the severity of the disease, and for comparison with postoperative ultrasound values on follow-up examinations.

Final diagnosis: PDA. Although this is a severe case, successful treatment can be achieved by surgical placement of a ligature or constricting band around the PDA, or an intracardiac catheter-placed occluding coil.

CASE 1.3

1 What are your radiographic findings? The cardiac silhouette is moderately enlarged with a globoid shape. The caudal vena cava is also large. Pleural fissure lines are not seen but there is the impression of reduced cranial abdominal serosal detail.

2 What is your radiographic diagnosis? Pericardial effusion is the most probable diagnosis. The impression of lack of abdominal detail suggests the potential for right-sided heart failure and ascites. Other possible differential diagnoses include: dilated cardiomyopathy (DCM), tricuspid dysplasia, or congenital peritoneopericardial hernia.

The physical examination makes tricuspid dysplasia less likely due to lack of a heart murmur. In cases of DCM, the left atrium is usually enlarged and quite evident radiographically, making DCM less likely than pericardial effusion in this case as the left atrium cannot be seen due to its location within the pericardial sac and silhouetting with the pericardial fluid. Note how in this case of pericardial effusion, the base of the heart is not abnormally shaped. DCM patients will usually show radiographic evidence of heart failure (left-sided or both left and right-sided) at the time of clinical presentation. Peritoneopericardial hernia is usually asymptomatic.

The enlarged caudal vena cava, although a nonspecific finding, supports a diagnosis of pericardial effusion, as does the impression of ascites. This is due to elevated central venous pressure, which occurs when pericardial effusion reaches a threshold and impedes right atrial filling. Both of these findings would also be expected to occur with heart failure from tricuspid dysplasia.

3 Is additional imaging needed? Echocardiography to confirm the diagnosis of pericardial effusion. An ultrasound-guided pericardiocentesis should be performed and the heart carefully examined to search for a common etiology of pericardial effusion, such as a right atrial tumor (hemangiosarcoma, common in German Shepherd Dogs) or a heart base tumor (aortic bony tumor, chemodectoma). The abdomen could also be scanned to verify the presence or absence of fluid and to search for concurrent disease, such as hemangiosarcoma of the spleen.

CASE 1.4

1 What are your radiographic findings? Multiple small to moderate-sized soft tissue nodules are seen throughout the pulmonary parenchyma, partially obscuring the margin of the cardiac silhouette, pulmonary blood vessels, caudal vena cava, and aorta. Incidental findings include thoracolumbar ventral spondylosis deformans and shoulder degenerative joint disease.

2 What is your radiographic diagnosis? Widespread pulmonary metastases.

3 Are any additional radiographs needed? A three-view examination of the thorax is often made to thoroughly assess the pulmonary parenchyma; however, this is not necessary in this case given the severity of the radiographic lesions.

Final diagnosis: Cytology of the liver and lung nodules, obtained with ultrasound guidance, was diagnostic for hepatocellular carcinoma with lung metastasis.

CASE 1.5

1 What are your radiographic findings? The pulmonary arteries are markedly enlarged, torturous, and blunted. Note the pulmonary veins are not affected. A mild interstitial pattern is present, particularly in the caudal lung lobes, obscuring vascular margin clarity. The cardiac silhouette is within normal limits.

2 What is your radiographic diagnosis? Severe pulmonary arterial enlargement/pulmonary hypertension. Differential diagnosis: heartworm disease, chronic interstitial lung disease, idiopathic interstitial fibrosis. This patient was negative for heartworm disease.

Final diagnosis: Pulmonary hypertension. Note how the enlarged pulmonary arteries when seen end-on appear as 'nodules' and could be misinterpreted as metastatic lung disease on casual observation of the images. In most cases with pulmonary arteries this large, there is concurrent main pulmonary artery and right ventricular enlargement radiographically.

CASE 1.6

1 What are your radiographic findings? There is an increase in soft tissue opacity in the right caudal lung lobe. Air bronchograms can be seen on the dorsoventral view and the pulmonary blood vessels are being silhouetted by the abnormal lung opacity; this contrasts nicely with the normally aerated left caudal lung in which the pulmonary blood vessels are easily identified and the bronchi are not as readily visible. The cardiac silhouette and pulmonary vasculature appear normal, as does the remainder of the lung.

2 What is your radiographic diagnosis? Right caudal lobar alveolar infiltrate (consolidation). The most likely differential diagnoses in this case include: noncardiogenic pulmonary edema, hemorrhage, lobar pneumonia.

3 Are any additional radiographic views needed? No.

Final diagnosis: Noncardiogenic pulmonary edema. This patient had chewed on an electrical cord and been electrocuted. Other differential diagnoses for noncardiogenic pulmonary edema include drowning and neurologic disease such as head trauma or seizures.

Comment: Most cases of electrical cord bite result in more profound, radiographically evident pulmonary edema, classically within the caudal lung lobes. Curiously, in this case the consolidated right caudal lung cannot be visualized with confidence on the left lateral view (as you would expect). Note that the right caudal pulmonary blood vessels are being effaced (silhouetted) by the edema within the interstitial space.

This case illustrates the importance of critical evaluation of radiographs and applying with confidence a few of the most basic principles of image interpretation (silhouette sign, air bronchograms).

CASE 1.7

1 What are your radiographic findings? There is gas dilation of the esophagus throughout its entire thoracic length. Ventrally located areas of alveolar pulmonary infiltrate are present in the left cranial lung lobe, both the cranial and caudal subsegments. These can be seen cranial to and overlying the heart on the right lateral view. On the dorsoventral view, these infiltrates are seen as an interstitial infiltrate, partially obscuring the pulmonary blood vessels and left cardiac margin. Note the lobar margin on the right lateral view, demarcating the consolidated left caudal lobe subsegment from normally aerated left caudal lung. It is difficult to identify lung pathology on the left lateral view. The trachea is ventrally depressed and the aorta is more conspicuous than normal.

2 What is your radiographic diagnosis? Megaesophagus with aspiration pneumonia.

Comment: The right middle lung lobe is the lung lobe most commonly affected in cases of aspiration pneumonia; therefore, this case is a bit unusual in that the right middle lung lobe is only minimally affected. The distribution in this case is typical for aspiration pneumonia as the ventral aspect of the lung lobes is most commonly diseased due to gravitational distribution. Careful assessment of lung overlying the heart is critical in identifying mild cases of pneumonia; infiltrates are more easily seen because of the summation effects of the heart. On dorsoventral or ventrodorsal views, the ventral-most lung pathology may be hidden by the midline structures, further emphasizing the importance of looking 'through the heart' into the lung on the lateral views and obtaining both right and left lateral views in these cases.

Note the ventral depression of the trachea, caused by the enlarged esophagus. This is a reliable radiographic finding that there is an enlarged esophagus. In many cases, the enlarged esophagus is not as readily apparent as this case illustrates. Also, the descending aorta is more apparent than normal, due to the air-filled esophagus adjacent to it.

Final diagnosis: Myasthenia gravis.

CASE 1.8

1 **What are your radiographic findings?** An alveolar pattern (consolidation) is present within the right middle lung lobe. This is best seen on the left lateral projection as increased soft tissue opacity and the presence of air bronchograms overlying the cardiac silhouette. This is also easily seen on the ventrodorsal projection as a triangular-shaped soft tissue opacity with effacement (silhouetting) of the right cardiac border. Note the striking appearance of the caudal margin of the consolidated right middle lung lobe against the aerated cranial margin of the right caudal lung lobe, termed a lobar sign. The rest of the lung lobes are normal. The cardiac silhouette is within normal limits. There is no indication of a dilated esophagus.

2 **What is your radiographic diagnosis?** Bronchopneumonia.

Comment: This case illustrates the effects of recumbency on lung evaluation. Note that on the right lateral view, the severely consolidated right middle lung disease is not very apparent, yet it is striking on the left lateral view. This is because the dependent lung is less aerated, becoming more soft tissue in opacity. This results in less contrast with the diseased lung (silhouette sign), making it very difficult to detect. Conversely, note how well the lobar consolidation is seen on the left lateral view, the nondependent lung, where the normal portions of the right middle lung are well inflated and thus provide good contrast.

CASE 1.9

1 **What are your radiographic findings?** An increase in soft tissue opacity is present bilaterally within the thoracic cavity. The cardiac silhouette is partially silhouetted (effaced) by the soft tissue opacity, especially on the dorsoventral view. A pleural fissure line is present on the dorsoventral projection between the right cranial and right middle lung lobes. On the lateral view, there is retraction of the ventral lung margin, creating a 'leafing' appearance. Pulmonary blood vessels are easily visualized. There is good abdominal serosal detail.

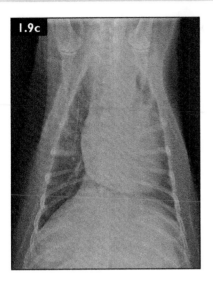

1.9c

2 **What is your radiographic diagnosis?** Moderate pleural effusion.

3 **Are additional radiographic projections needed?** A ventrodorsal projection should be obtained to better visualize the cardiac silhouette (**Fig. 1.9c**). Redistribution of pleural fluid on the ventrodorsal view allows the lungs to 'float' up and around the heart, allowing assessment of cardiac size. In this case, fissure lines are present. The cardiac silhouette is slightly larger than expected, with increased width and cardiophrenic contact. The etiology of the pleural fluid is not determined from the radiographic study.

Comment: The final diagnosis was made from ultrasound examination of the heart and cytologic analysis of the fluid. Note that a smaller amount of pericardial fluid does not render the cardiac silhouette a globoid structure.

Final diagnosis: Idiopathic pleural effusion and pericardial effusion.

CASE 1.10

1 **What are your radiographic findings?** The cardiac silhouette is enlarged, being both too tall and too wide. On the dorsoventral view, the left atrium is enlarged, extending to the right of midline, giving the appearance of biatrial enlargement, which is also known as the 'valentine' appearance. The right cranial pulmonary vasculature is mildly enlarged, although symmetrical. A very mild increase in soft tissue opacity is present in the right caudal pulmonary parenchyma. Occasional bronchial markings are identified diffusely throughout the pulmonary parenchyma. Incidentally, a spherical metal pellet is present along the apex of the heart.

2 **What is your radiographic diagnosis?** Cardiomegaly, including left atrial enlargement; mild right caudal interstitial pulmonary pattern, most consistent with mild pulmonary edema and early congestive heart failure.

3 **Is additional imaging needed?** Echocardiography could be performed to further evaluate the heart. Additionally, an abdominal ultrasound to determine if the cat has a caudal aortic thrombus, which is seen in patients with hypertrophic cardiomyopathy.

Final diagnosis: Hypertrophic cardiomyopathy.

CASE 1.11

1 What are your radiographic findings? There is a diffuse but heterogeneous increase in soft tissue opacity of the thorax, partially obscuring the cardiac silhouette. Lung lobe margins are rounded and easily identified and thin pleural fissures are seen. On the left lateral view, the dorsal surface of a caudal lung lobe can be seen retracted well away from the dorsal pleural surface and traced along the diaphragm margin, indicating an pneumothorax. The cranial lung surface is also seen, as is a widened fissure between them. On the right lateral view, a more focal area of soft tissue opacity is seen in the caudodorsal thorax characterized by a thin curved caudal border and irregular areas of more focal soft tissue opacity; this is felt to be located in the left caudal lung based on its nonvisualization on the left lateral view and a similar appearing area within the left caudal lung on the ventrodorsal view. There is abnormal soft tissue opacity located in the pleural space, with an especially prominent area noted adjacent to the left caudal lung margin on the ventrodorsal view. There are numerous round gas 'pockets' noted on the lateral views, over the cardiac silhouette and sternum. The majority of the pulmonary blood vessels are identified but the presence of multifocal pulmonary infiltrates cannot be ruled out. Although partially obscured, the cardiac silhouette is within normal limits, based on normal tracheal location and overall impression of a proper size and cardiothoracic ratio.

2 What is your radiographic diagnosis? Heterogeneous pleural effusion, mild left-sided pneumothorax and suspected left caudal lung lobe mass. Differential diagnosis: the two most reasonable differential diagnoses are infectious pyothorax secondary to a pulmonary abscess and widespread thoracic neoplasia.

Comment: This is a visually overwhelming case radiographically and perfectly illustrates the importance of utilizing basic radiographic principles to work your way through the interpretation. It should be noted here that identification of pulmonary disease in the face of pleural effusion is difficult and sometimes a reliable assessment cannot be made regarding the pulmonary parenchyma; observation of pulmonary blood vessels is paramount, since the lungs will appear more opaque due to the overlying soft tissue opacity of the pleural fluid (summation effect).

Final diagnosis: At surgery, an abscess was found in the left caudal lung lobe secondary to a rose thorn. A pyothorax was also present. The patient recovered completely.

CASE 1.12

1 What are your radiographic findings? A severe interstitial to alveolar pattern is present in all lung lobes. The majority of the pulmonary blood vessels are silhouetting with this infiltrate, except the largest cranial lobar vessels near the hilus.

Both the arteries and vein are enlarged. Note that the caudal vena cava and descending aorta cannot be seen because of the pulmonary infiltrates. The cardiac silhouette can only be partially visualized due to silhouetting of its margins with the pulmonary infiltrates; however, it does appear large based on the dorsoventral view and the position of the dorsally deviated trachea on the lateral view. On the dorsoventral view, there is separation of the lung margins from the parietal pleural surface by soft tissue opacity, especially caudally, and pleural fissure lines are seen separating the lung lobes. Rounded pleural fissures are also noted on the lateral view, separating the caudal from middle lobes. These latter findings indicate the presence of pleural effusion. Abdominal detail appears normal.

2 What is your radiographic diagnosis? Left-sided congestive heart failure (pulmonary edema and pleural effusion).

3 Is further imaging needed? Echocardiography would be recommended.

   Final diagnosis: Hypertrophic cardiomyopathy (HCM).

Comment: HCM in cats often leads to both pulmonary edema and pleural effusion, unlike the dog in which pleural effusion is a sign of right-sided heart failure. Both pulmonary arterial and venous enlargement are usually noted.

CASE 1.13

1 What are your radiographic findings? The cardiac silhouette is enlarged, both too tall on the lateral view and elongated on the dorsoventral view. There is rounding of the left ventricular apex and the left ventricle is large based on the dorsoventral view. There is loss of the cranial cardiac waist (lateral view) with a small soft tissue bulge. A triangular soft tissue opacity is present in the cranial thorax on midline and to the left, indicative of the thymus. The pulmonary parenchyma and vessels are within normal limits, as they can be easily seen on the dorsoventral view.

2 What is your radiographic diagnosis? Left-sided cardiomegaly and cranial cardiac waist enlargement. The primary differential diagnosis is subaortic stenosis.

   Final diagnosis: Subaortic stenosis

3 Is further imaging needed? Echocardiography to confirm the diagnosis and obtain baseline data and for prognostication. In this case, the subaortic stenosis was severe. This is suspected on the radiographs because the cardiac enlargement is quite severe given the very young age of the patient.

Comment: The elongated cardiac silhouette on the dorsoventral view is diagnostic for left ventricular enlargement. The increased soft tissue of the cranial cardiac waist is usually indicative of aortic arch enlargement, pulmonic outflow enlargement, or an enlarged right auricle. These can be differentiated from one another based on the dorsoventral/ventrodorsal view; the aortic arc enlargement is located on midline, the main pulmonary artery is enlarged at the 1 o'clock position, while the right atrium/auricle will show itself at the 9–11 o'clock location. The thymus is located in the cranial mediastinum and will be evident in most puppies. Note that the cranial mediastinum crosses midline to the left. Keep this in mind when reviewing adult dogs with a mediastinal mass; thymomas and other cranial mediastinal masses often will extend to the left, a clue as to their origin.

CASE 1.14

1 What are your radiographic findings? The cardiac silhouette is greatly enlarged. It is too tall and elongated, the trachea is elevated dorsally and nearly parallels the spine. The heart is too wide as well, being greater than four intercostal spaces. The caudal cardiac waist is large and protrudes caudally, indicating a greatly enlarged left atrium. There is focal enlargement at the 1 o'clock position on the dorsoventral view, indicating an enlarged main pulmonary artery (MPA). There is also a focal enlargement of the proximal descending aorta seen just medial to the enlarged MPA. The pulmonary blood vessels are moderately enlarged and matched, the arteries being equal in size to the veins. While the pulmonary blood vessels are easily identified, some of the larger ones in the perihilar region have indistinct margins, indicating a mild interstitial pulmonary infiltrate.

2 What is your radiographic diagnosis? Left-sided cardiomegaly and pulmonary overcirculation, consistent with a left-to-right patent ductus arteriosus; suspect early (mild) pulmonary edema (heart failure).

Final diagnosis: Patent ductus arteriosus.

CASE 1.15

1 What are your radiographic findings? The cardiac silhouette is markedly enlarged, causing dorsal deviation of the trachea. It is too wide and too tall, with an increase in the cardiothoracic ratio. There are multiple gas-filled tubular structures summating with the

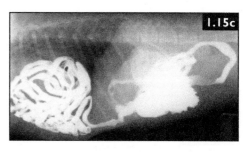

cardiac silhouette, representing small intestine. The diameter of the intestinal segments is within normal limits. There are only six sternebrae. There is no dorsal mesothelial remnant.

2 What is your radiographic diagnosis? Congenital peritoneopericardial diaphragmatic hernia (PPDH) containing small intestine.

3 Is additional imaging needed? Cardiac ultrasound examination or positive contrast peritoneography may be helpful. This gastrointestinal barium contrast radiograph (**Fig. 1.15c**) shows small intestine contained within the pericardial sac. However, it was not necessary in this case to make the correct diagnosis.

Comment: PPDHs are always congenital and usually an incidental finding in cats and dogs. Associated sternebral abnormalities and a dorsal mesothelial remnant may be present in these cases. The hernia is not always surgically corrected unless an intestinal obstruction occurs within the herniated small intestines or liver or fat is incarcerated and compromised. The 'globoid' appearance of the cardiac silhouette can clearly be differentiated from the other three differential diagnoses by the presence of the gas-filled intestinal loops. If they were only fluid filled, other imaging, such as a cardiac ultrasound examination, or positive contrast peritoneography, would be needed to give a definitive diagnosis. Note that unless a PPDH contains bowel, a negative barium study may be misleading, as in many cases the PPDH contains falciform fat or liver, not intestine. In the case of falciform fat, the heart may be visualized because it is surrounded by less opaque fat. Radiography of the abdomen may show a lack of normal structures, such as small intestines in this case, or an altered gastric axis if liver is herniated.

This is a good case to illustrate the use of the term 'cardiac silhouette' instead of the word 'heart'. Cardiac silhouette is used to include the composite radiographic image of the heart, pericardium, and pericardial space. In this example, the heart itself is not enlarged, so to say the heart is big is misleading at best.

CASE 1.16

1 What are your radiographic findings? There is a large, spherical, well-circumscribed mass within the right caudal lung lobe. Internally, it is heterogeneous, having aerated areas interspersed with consolidated lung. The remaining thoracic structures are normal.

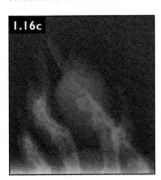

2 What is your radiographic diagnosis? Cavitary, complex right caudal pulmonary mass and lytic third phalanx of the right hind third phalange. The most probable diagnosis is a primary lung tumor (bronchogenic adenocarcinoma) with metastasis to the digits.

3 Are additional radiographs needed? Radiography of the swollen left hind toe should be performed (**Fig. 1.16c**). There is soft tissue swelling of the third digit with bony lysis of the third phalanx of this digit.

Final diagnosis: Bronchogenic carcinoma with metastasis to the left hind third digit.

CASE 1.17

1 What are your radiographic findings?
There is a large focus of increased soft tissue opacity containing gas within the dorsal caudal thorax just left of midline. The cardiac silhouette and pulmonary vasculature are within normal limits. The spine is within normal limits.

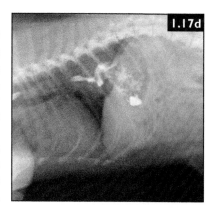

2 What is your radiographic diagnosis? Large soft tissue, gas-containing mass in the caudal thorax near midline. Differential diagnoses include: a sliding (intermittent) gastric hiatal hernia (fixed or sliding/intermittent), an esophageal mass, a pulmonary mass, or an abscess within the caudal mediastinum.

3 Is additional imaging needed? Differentiation of these potential diagnoses can be challenging. In this case, an esophagram was performed, which confirmed a hiatal hernia. In this static image (**Fig. 1.17d**), obtained during a dynamic fluoroscopic examination, the stomach is partially herniated into the thorax; it contains barium, delineating gastric rugal folds, and represents the structure seen on the survey thoracic films. Whether or not the hiatal hernia is responsible for the clinical presentation is uncertain, but is probably an incidental and unrelated finding in this case.

Final diagnosis: Hiatal hernia.

Comment: Sliding hiatal hernias are not uncommon and usually are considered an incidental finding. They can be breed related and congenital, such as in the Shar Pei and English Bulldog. However, they can be a manifestation of increased respiratory effort, as may be seen with feline asthma, restrictive lung disease or upper airway disease.

CASE 1.18

1 What are your radiographic findings? There is abnormal soft tissue opacity dorsal to the cardiac silhouette at the level of T3–6, displacing the trachea rightward and ventrally. The carina of the trachea is displaced caudally to the level of the seventh ribs, positioned at the level of the caudal heart base, indicative of right ventricular enlargement. The cardiac silhouette is round and enlarged. There is a small round soft tissue opacity within the pulmonary parenchyma dorsal to the second sternebra, seen best on the left lateral view.

2 What is your radiographic diagnosis? Perihilar heart-based mass. The primary differential diagnoses are mediastinal lymphadenopathy and a heart base tumor. Also suspect a pulmonary nodule, most likely metastatic disease. Cardiomegaly.

Comment: There are two basic forms of heart base neoplasia; right atrial hemangiosarcoma and aortic body tumors (chemodectomas). Right atrial enlargement is rarely seen as a discrete mass, usually causing pericardial hemorrhage and thus hidden from view. Aortic body tumors may or may not cause hemorrhage into the pericardial sac. Hilar or mediastinal lymphadenopathy can occur from neoplasia, lymphosarcoma being the most common heart base form. Lymphadenopathy from granulomatous infectious processes are less common but do occur secondary to fungal or anaerobic disease. Recall that the hilar lymph nodes reside between the left and right cranial lobar bronchi and between the caudal bronchi. In this case, the trachea is displaced markedly to the right, an unusual finding for hilar lymphadenopathy, making cranial mediastinal lymph node enlargement a better differential diagnosis than hilar nodal enlargement.

In addition to cardiac ultrasound, thoracic computed tomography (CT) could be used to better delineate the extent of the disease and assess the lungs for pulmonary nodules not seen on the thoracic radiographs. CT would also be the procedure of choice to obtain a fine needle aspirate or tissue biopsy, although the location makes sampling a moderately risky procedure. Fluoroscopy could also be used to obtain a cytologic or histologic diagnosis.

Final diagnosis: Echocardiography showed a large infiltrating mass surrounding the aorta and pulmonary artery, causing compression of the right pulmonary artery and occluding blood flow into the atria. Atrial enlargement was responsible for the enlarged cardiac silhouette.

CASE 1.19

1 What are your radiographic findings? There is an increase in soft tissue opacity within the right pleural space, which is very irregular in outline. The cardiac silhouette is markedly shifted to the right, as no heart shadow can be seen in the left hemithorax. All of the lung lobes show some degree of volume loss. The cranial lung lobes are completely collapsed, as is the right middle lobe. The right caudal lung is reduced in size, is very rounded in shape, and has a mottled soft tissue opacity interspersed with aerated parenchyma. Note the large pulmonary artery and vein to this lobe. The left caudal lung lobe is faintly seen retracted away from the parietal pleural surface, having lost perhaps one-half of its volume; it is rounded in shape similar to the right caudal lung. Along the left hemithoax and on midline caudally there is free pleural air. The other lung lobes contain an increase in soft tissue opacity. There is little difference in the appearance between the ventrodorsal and dorsoventral views, indicating trapped or loculated pleural fluid, or soft tissue thickening of the pleura. As an incidental finding, the aortic arch is prominent on the ventrodorsal and dorsoventral views, enhanced by the pneumothorax and the mediastinal shift.

2 What is your radiographic diagnosis? Tension pneumothorax, left-sided; pleural disease, primarily right sided; complete collapse of the cranial and middle lung lobes, partial collapse of the other lung lobes; suspect right caudal lung lobe pathology. The etiology for these findings is not clear from the radiographic study. Differential diagnoses include: ruptured right caudal lung pathology (abscess, neoplasia), pyothorax and resultant sequelae, thoracic neoplasia.

Comment: This is a challenging case radiographically, with a multitude of findings. The mediastinal shift to the right in face of the left-sided pneumothorax indicates a positive intrathoracic pressure, since with a nontension pneumothorax the heart and mediastinum should shift toward the side of the pneumothorax. Tension pneumothorax is an emergency; if the pressure becomes too great, the lung will completely collapse, becoming nonfunctional. Intervention to relieve the tension pneumothorax is indicated.
   Final diagnosis: Fine needle aspirates of the right-sided pleural disease proved diagnostic, yielding neoplastic cells (origin undetermined).

CASE 1.20

1 What are your radiographic findings? There is diffuse, thin, bronchial wall mineralization seen as thin parallel ('tram lines') and end-on ('doughnuts') airways present throughout the lungs. There are also multiple small mineral focal opacities present throughout the lungs.
2 What is your radiographic diagnosis? Bronchial wall mineralization may represent the consequences of chronic bronchitis. Pulmonary osteomas (pulmonary osseous metaplasia) are an incidental finding.

Comment: There is some debate as to whether or not bronchial wall mineralization actually occurs. The airways in this patient are easily identified, but they do taper normally as they branch into the periphery (i.e. bronchiectasis is not present). This is a very nonspecific finding and may be unrelated to the history of cough. The majority of bronchitis cases do not manifest radiographically.
   Pulmonary osteomas are small (several millimeters) benign islands of mineralization just under the visceral pleural surface of the lung. They can be a result of prior infectious disease such as parasite migration, although in most cases the etiology is undetermined. They can be recognized by their small size and the fact that they are mineral opacities; if they were soft tissue nodules, they would not be seen radiographically, too small to be resolved on a thoracic radiograph, even a digitally acquired one. Rarely, metastatic osteosarcoma can manifest as small osseous nodules, but in almost all cases there is known osteosarcoma identified in the appendicular or axial skeleton.

CASE 1.21

1 What are your radiographic findings? Cardiomegaly is present, as the cardiac silhouette is too tall and long. In particular the right atrium is enlarged, seen as an abnormal soft tissue bulge in the 9–11 o'clock position on the dorsoventral view. The area of the right ventricle is not enlarged (9–6 o'clock). On the right lateral view, the enlarged right auricle is seen as a discrete curved soft tissue margin over the cardiac silhouette. The pulmonary parenchyma and vasculature are within normal limits, but the caudal vena cava is very large and 'kinked' on the lateral view.

2 What is your radiographic diagnosis? Right atrial enlargement with no evidence of heart failure. The congenital cardiac disease tricuspid dysplasia is the most likely diagnosis.

3 Is additional imaging needed? Echocardiography.

Final diagnosis: Echocardiography of this patient showed tricuspid valvular dysplasia, a markedly enlarged right atrium, and a hypoplastic pulmonary outflow tract.

CASE 1.22

1 What are your radiographic findings? A poorly-defined, unstuctured (i.e. not nodular), multifocal interstitial pattern is present in the caudal lung lobes. The pulmonary vasculature and cardiac silhouette are within normal limits.

2 What is your radiographic diagnosis? Diffuse unstructured interstitial pulmonary infiltrate, nonspecific for etiology. Primary differential diagnoses include inflammatory or infectious disease. The pattern is atypical for heart failure and pulmonary edema, and it is also not typical of noncardiogenic edema, pulmonary hemorrhage, or neoplasia.

Final diagnosis: A bronchoalveolar lavage was performed and a diagnosis of *Paragonimus* infection made.

CASE 1.23

1 What are your radiographic findings? There is an overall increase in opacity to the thorax, due primarily to soft tissue opacity present within the pleural space. Retraction of the lung lobes (leafing) and pleural fissure lines is noted. There is also an increase in opacity of the caudodorsal lung fields (interstitial infiltrate). The pulmonary blood vessel margins are partially obscured, but larger vessels can still be seen and are enlarged and mismatched; the veins are larger than the arteries. The caudal vena cava and aorta cannot be seen. The margins of the heart are partially obscured by both pleural and pulmonary soft tissue opacities. Still, the cardiac silhouette is generally and severely enlarged. It is too wide and tall with dorsal tracheal displacement. There is an enlarged caudal cardiac waist and increased opacity with mainstem bronchial splaying on the dorsoventral view. The ventrodorsal view shows redistribution of the pleural soft tissue opacity, indicating freely moveable pleural effusion. The ventrodorsal view allows better assessment of the enlarged cardiac silhouette. The right atrium is noted to be enlarged on this view.

2 What is your radiographic diagnosis? Generalized cardiomegaly with biventricular failure, characterized by pulmonary edema, pleural effusion. The primary differential diagnosis is dilated cardiomyopathy (DCM), common in the Doberman Pinscher dog.

Final diagnosis: Echocardiography confirmed DCM as the diagnosis.

CASE 1.24

1 What are your radiographic findings? There is a diffuse increase in soft tissue opacity throughout the lung. Careful inspection of the pulmonary infiltrate clearly shows an airway distribution of the increased lung opacity. This can be classified as a severe, diffuse bronchial or peribronchial pattern. The bronchi appear to taper properly as they extend to the periphery of the lung. Large areas of consolidating pulmonary infiltrates are not present, although at the terminal portions of some airways there is the suggestion of mild focal consolidation. The lungs are hyperinflated, indicated by how far caudal the diaphragm is positioned on both views. Because of this, the heart appears relatively small.

2 What is your radiographic diagnosis? Severe bronchial disease characterized by both bronchial and peribronchial infiltrates, without bronchopneumonia or bronchiectasis. The primary differential diagnosis is an allergic bronchitis.

Comment: In this case, the bronchial walls are evident as thin soft tissue markings, but more striking is the thick peribronchial interstitial infiltrate, causing both 'donuts' and 'tramlines' as well as a reduction in pulmonary vascular margin detail. The hyperinflated state may be transitory or indicate air-trapping. An expiratory thoracic radiograph can verify or refute the latter.

The radiographic difference between a bronchial pattern and a peribronchial pattern can be difficult to ascertain in some cases. A peribronchial pattern is most commonly associated with allergic, infectious, or inflammatory lower airway disease (bronchitis), although some cases of cardiogenic pulmonary edema can have a preferential peribronchial distribution, especially in cats. Bronchial patterns, characterized by mineralization of airway walls and/or bronchiectasis, are usually associated with mucociliary disorders or chronic aspiration pneumonia.

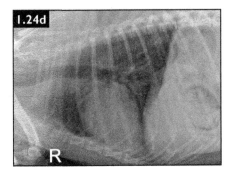

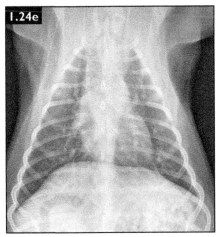

Final diagnosis: In this case, a bronchoalveolar lavage was performed. Cytology showed an increased percentage of eosinophils consistent with eosinophilic bronchopneumopathy, a sterile process related to a hypersensitivity reaction. This condition is known as pulmonary infiltrates with eosinophils (PIE). Circulating eosinophilia is a part of this disease process.

Radiographs obtained following 1 week of corticosteroid therapy are shown (Figs. 1.24d, e). The peribronchial interstitial infiltrate has resolved; however, a mild residual bronchial pattern is still present, as the airway walls, while thin, are quite easily seen. Note how much better the vascular detail is. The patient has responded well to therapy. It remains to be seen if the bronchial pattern will resolve, represents permanent damage to the airways, or is an incidental finding.

CASE 1.25

1 What are your radiographic findings? The cardiac silhouette is too wide on the dorsoventral view due to an increase in size of the right side of the heart; it has the appearance of a reverse 'D'. Note the left heart is straight, the apex small by comparison. Although subtle, the lateral views confirm right ventricular enlargement; the location of the carina relative to the heart is displaced caudally, indicating right ventricular enlargement. There is mild enlargement of the main pulmonary artery, seen at 1–2 o'clock on the dorsoventral view, corresponding to mild increased soft tissue opacity of the cranial cardiac waist on the lateral view. The pulmonary vasculature is mildly decreased in size, but the arteries and veins are of similar size. The pulmonary parenchyma is within normal limits.

2 What is your radiographic diagnosis? Congenital cardiac anomaly, most consistent with pulmonic stenosis (PS). The other differential diagnosis is a tetralogy of Fallot (TOF), but the descending aorta is easily visualized and properly positioned.

3 Is additional imaging needed? Echocardiography and angiocardiography. A single, still image frame from a fluoroscopic angiocardiographic study of the right ventricular outflow tract and main pulmonary artery is shown (**Fig. 1.25d**). A catheter has been placed into the right ventricle via the jugular vein (access via the cranial vena cava, right atrium, and right atrioventricular valve). (**Note:** Fluoroscopic images are usually displayed black-on-white, the reverse of a radiographic image.)

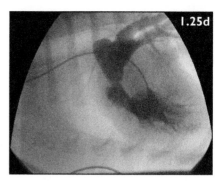

Comment: The angiocardiogram shows a valvular stenosis, seen as the constriction in the right ventricular outflow tract. There is a post-stenotic dilation present just distal to this. The dilated main pulmonary artery noted on the dorsoventral view and the increased opacity along the cranial waist of the heart is due to this dilation. There is mild enlargement of the main pulmonary artery, seen at 1 to 2 o'clock, on the DV view. The pulmonary vasculature is mildly decreased in size. The right ventricular wall is markedly thickened, noted radiographically as right heart enlargement.

Small pulmonary blood vessels can occur when right ventricular outflow is severely compromised, as in severe PS. The differential diagnosis of TOF is included because two of the components of TOF overlap those of PS (recall that PS, right ventricular hypertrophy, ventricular septal defect, and overriding aorta comprise the anomalies of TOF). It was noted that the aortic arch and descending aorta were normally located in this case, making TOF less likely.

Final diagnosis: Pulmonic stenosis.

CASE 1.26

1 **What are your radiographic findings?** The cardiac silhouette is severely enlarged and misshapen. It is shifted to the right (dextro-positioned). There is increased diaphragmatic and sternal contact on the lateral view. The apex of the heart is large and rounded. The pulmonary arteries and veins are very enlarged but matched in size. Obvious pulmonary parenchyma disease is not identified.

2 **What is your radiographic diagnosis?** Severe cardiomegaly and overcirculation, diagnostic for congenital heart disease with a left-to-right shunt. Congenital heart defects such as ventricular septal defect and patent ductus arteriosus are the most common causes of left-to-right shunts.

3 **Is additional imaging needed?** Echocardiography.

Comment: Dextro-positioning of the heart usually indicates left-sided cardiac enlargement though it can be an incidental finding.

Final diagnosis: Ventricular septal defect.

CASE 1.27

1 What are your radiographic findings? The cardiac silhouette and pulmonary vasculature are reduced in size. The pulmonary parenchyma is within normal limits. There are multiple, pinpoint mineral opaque foci within the peripheral lung fields, consistent with pulmonary osteomata.

2 What is your radiographic diagnosis? Reduced size of cardiovascular structures. The most likely differential diagnosis in this case is dehydration, as the dog is having difficulty drinking with the neurologic deficits. Other considerations for a small heart include Addison's disease and hypovolemia or shock.

CASE 1.28

1 What are your radiographic findings? Increased soft tissue opacity is present diffusely throughout the right caudal lung lobe, silhouetting with the diaphragm and caudal aspect of the cardiac silhouette. The remainder of the pulmonary parenchyma and the cardiovascular structures are within normal limits. An endotracheal tube is noted.

2 What is your radiographic diagnosis? Focal, right caudal lung lobe alveolar pattern. The primary differential diagnosis in this case is pneumonia. A pulmonary tumor is considered less likely given the cat's age.

Final diagnosis: Bronchopneumonia secondary to grass awn inhalation.

CASE 1.29

1 What are your radiographic findings? A focal, round soft tissue opacity is present cranial to the cardiac silhouette, dorsal to the 1st to 3rd sternebrae, and along midline, likely within the cranial mediastinum. The esophagus is moderately dilated with gas throughout the thoracic cavity. The cardiac silhouette, pulmonary vasculature, and pulmonary parenchyma are within normal limits.

2 What is your radiographic diagnosis? Megaesophagus, small cranial mediastinal mass.

Comment: Given the megaesophagus, the most likely differential diagnosis for the cranial mediastinal mass is a thymoma. Myasthenia gravis is a paraneoplastic syndrome associated with thymomas, which can cause a focal or generalized megaesophagus.

CASE 1.30

1 What are your radiographic findings? The cardiac silhouette is enlarged. On the lateral view, a large bulge is present in the cardiac silhouette, in the region of the right atrium; however, right atrial enlargement cannot be appreciated on the orthogonal view. On the ventrodorsal view, the cardiac silhouette appears elongated with rounding of the apex, suggestive of left ventricular enlargement. The pulmonary vasculature and pulmonary parenchyma are within normal limits.

2 What is your radiographic diagnosis? Cardiomegaly, with suspected right atrial enlargement.

3 Is additional imaging needed? Yes, echocardiography.

Comment: Right atrial enlargement is not definitively identified radiographically very often. The primary differential diagnoses for right atrial enlargement include tricuspid dysplasia or a right atrial mass.

Final diagnosis: Right atrial mass.

CASE 1.31

1 What are your radiographic findings? The cardiac silhouette is markedly enlarged, with dorsal displacement of the trachea and increased width. The left atrium is markedly enlarged, visualized caudal to the carina on the lateral view and between the splayed mainstem bronchi on the dorsoventral view. The left mainstem bronchus is narrowed by the severely enlarged left atrium (lateral projection). Additionally, the left auricle is enlarged, visualized at the 2–3 o'clock position on the dorsoventral view. The pulmonary vasculature and pulmonary parenchyma are within normal limits.

2 What is your radiographic diagnosis? Marked left-sided cardiomegaly, with severe left atrial and auricular enlargement.

3 Is additional imaging needed? An echocardiogram would be recommended in this case to further evaluate the heart.

Comment: In an older, small dog, the most likely differential diagnosis is mitral insufficiency, secondary to mitral valve endocardiosis. Note how the left atrial enlargement is causing narrowing of the left mainstem bronchus. This is a common finding in cases of left atrial enlargement and likely associated with the cough in this patient.

CASE 1.32

1 What are your radiographic findings? There is a moderate diffuse bronchial pattern present throughout the pulmonary parenchyma. End-on airways are seen as round, air-filled soft tissue structures ('donuts'), while longitudinally oriented airways are seen as thin parallel lines ('tramlines'). The lungs are overly inflated on the lateral view, although they do not show severe overinflation on the dorsoventral view.

2 What is your radiographic diagnosis? Moderate bronchitis. This is most likely due to chronic feline asthma.

Comment: In feline asthma, there may be bronchial wall thickening, intraluminal mucus, and peribronchial migration of inflammatory cells (predominately plasmocytes and lymphocytes), which is seen collectively as airway thickening. Mucus bronchial plugs can lead to lung lobe collapse, especially the right middle lobe. Hyperinflation and air-trapping are additional commonly encountered radiographic manifestations of feline asthma. Finally, feline asthma may not manifest itself radiographically, as some patients have normal radiographs.

Hyperinflation is also one of the radiographic features of upper or lower airway disease in cats and it may be the only radiographic abnormality appreciated. Hyperinflation should be differentiated from air-trapping by comparing inspiratory and expiratory radiographs. With air-trapping, there is little or no difference in the degree of lung inflation. Other signs of hyperinflation include flattening or 'tenting' of the diaphragm, created by focal flattening of the diaphragm at sites of costal attachment. Hyperinflation can also be produced simply by the stress of the procedure or an underlying endocrinopathy (e.g. hyperthyroidism).

CASE 1.33

1 What are your radiographic findings? Patchy multifocal nodular interstitial infiltrate with poorly defined margins are present within all lung lobes. The pulmonary blood vessels are silhouetting with this infiltrate. The cardiac silhouette is normal.

2 What is your radiographic diagnosis? Severe, multifocal, patchy interstitial pulmonary pattern. Differential diagnoses include: pneumonia, with both hematogenous and inhalation routes considered, and neoplasia (e.g. metastatic carcinoma). *Toxoplasma*, *Mycoplasma*, and *Cryptococcus* are possible infectious etiologies for the pulmonary pattern in this cat.

Final diagnosis: *Mycoplasma* pneumonia. This diagnosis was obtained on an ultrasound-guided fine needle aspirate of a lung nodule. The cytology showed degenerative neutrophils and intracellular bacteria and the culture was positive for *Mycoplasma*.

CASE 1.34

1 What are your radiographic findings? There is a diffuse interstitial pattern present throughout the pulmonary parenchyma obscuring to some degree the pulmonary vascular markings. Close inspection of the pulmonary infiltrate shows the presence of very small nodules. There are several areas where the pulmonary infiltrate has begun to coalesce. The cardiovascular structures are within normal limits. The focal elevated intrathoracic trachea is probably a result of a hyperflexed head and neck, creating a 'kink'. There is no evidence of a mediastinal mass creating this.

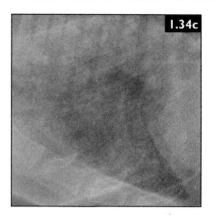

2 What is your radiographic diagnosis? Diffuse interstitial pulmonary pattern, both structured and unstructured with multiple very small nodules (**Fig. 1.34c**, close-up view of the cranioventral lung). The primary differential diagnosis in this case is diffuse pulmonary metastatic disease.

Final diagnosis: Hemangiosarcoma.

CASE 1.35

1 What are your radiographic findings? There is a focal increase in soft tissue opacity present dorsal to the 1st to 3rd sternebrae, corresponding to enlarged sternal lymph nodes. No abnormalities of the cardiovascular structures are appreciated. The pulmonary parenchyma is normal for a geriatric patient. A very mild increase in soft tissue density is identified within the ventral thorax, with mild rounding/leafing of the lung lobe margins on the lateral view. Note that the caudal-most thorax is not included on the ventrodorsal radiograph.

2 What is your radiographic diagnosis? Sternal lymphadenopathy and minimal pleural effusion.

Comment: Recall that the sternal lymph node(s) primarily receives lymphatic drainage from the abdominal surface of the diaphragm and cranial abdomen. Sternal lymph node enlargement is most often secondary to abdominal disease (e.g. inflammatory/infectious disease, metastatic disease) or systemic disease affecting the lymphatic system (e.g. lymphosarcoma, malignant histiocytosis).

Final diagnosis: Malignant histiocytosis, obtained by cytology of the sternal lymph node via ultrasound guidance.

CASE 1.36

1 What are your radiographic findings? A soft tissue mass is identified within the right mid-thorax, at the level of the right 4th to 6th ribs on the dorsoventral projection and overlying the caudal border of the cardiac silhouette on the lateral projection. Close inspection shows lysis of the 6th rib near its junction with the costal cartilage.

This is best appreciated when compared with the adjacent 5th and 7th rib ends. The pulmonary parenchyma and cardiovascular structures are normal.

2 What is your radiographic diagnosis? Expansile and destructive right 6th rib mass. The primary differential diagnosis is an aggressive osseous lesion, such as neoplasia (e.g. primary or metastatic neoplastic disease) or osteomyelitis.

Comment: Differentiating this rib mass from a mass of pulmonary origin is very difficult. The clue in this case is observation of the rib lysis. Rib lysis usually indicates a lesion of rib origin; it is unusual for a pulmonary mass to invade a rib. Without rib lysis, we would need to list a pulmonary mass and a rib mass as differential radiographic diagnoses.

Thoracic body wall masses often originate from the ribs (chondrosarcoma, osteosarcoma). In addition to radiology, ultrasound and computed tomography can be used to assess the degree of body wall involvement, including the ribs and lung, which is helpful in planning surgical resection. Guided biopsies of intrathoracic masses can also be obtained by using these modalities.

CASE 1.37

1 What are your radiographic findings? Increased soft tissue opacity, with rounded margins, is present in the perihilar region on the lateral view, causing ventral deviation of the caudal thoracic trachea and carina. On the ventrodorsal view, there is mild splaying of the mainstem bronchi by a soft tissue opacity. The remainder of the thorax is unremarkable.

2 What is your radiographic diagnosis? Perihilar lymphadenopathy.

Comment: Perihilar lymphadenopathy is difficult to detect radiographically, as the lymph nodes need to become large enough to identify them with confidence. If suspected, a computed tomography examination could be performed to confirm lymphadenopathy in this region. There are three tracheobronchial lymph nodes: the right, left and middle. The middle lymph node is located between the mainstem bronchi, along midline on the ventrodorsal view. The right lymph node is located to the right of the caudal tracheal and mainstem bronchus and the left is in a similar location on the left side. Lymphadenomegaly in this region can cause ventral deviation of the trachea, in comparison with left atrial enlargement, which elevates the caudal trachea dorsally. The most common causes of hilar lymph node enlargement are malignancies, such as lymphoma and histiocytic sarcoma, and fungal disease.

CASE 1.38

1 What are your radiographic findings? There is a patchy, diffuse increase in soft tissue opacity affecting nearly all the mid- to ventral lung, extending dorsally on the left. These areas are consolidated, with air bronchograms identified (an alveolar pattern). The caudodorsal lung is relatively spared. A focal nodule can be seen in the dorsal-most lung on the left lateral radiograph. The cardiac silhouette is obscured by the severe pulmonary infiltrates, as are many of the pulmonary blood vessels. It does not appear enlarged based on the lateral view. The tracheal diameter is greater than expected and is a reflection of increased respiratory effort.

2 **What is your radiographic diagnosis?** Severe, diffuse infiltrative pulmonary disease. Etiology cannot be determined from the radiographs. Differential diagnoses are numerous in this case and include: infectious disease, cardiogenic and noncardiogenic pulmonary edema, and hemorrhage.

Comment: Cardiac ultrasound would identify if heart failure was present, although unlikely in this case since a heart murmur, expected in most congenital cardiac anomalies, was not auscultated. A fine needle aspirate of the lung may prove to be diagnostic.

Final diagnosis: Toxoplasmosis, diagnosed at necropsy.

CASE 1.39

1 **What are your radiographic findings?** The right cranial and right middle bronchi are dilated. A moderate increase in soft tissue opacity is present in the ventral portions of the right cranial and right middle lung lobes, consistent with an alveolar pattern. The cardiovascular structures are within normal limits.

2 **What is your radiographic diagnosis?** Right cranial and right middle bronchiectasis and a ventrally distributed alveolar pulmonary pattern, diagnostic for pneumonia.

Final diagnosis: Bronchopneumonia and bronchiectasis.

Comment: Bronchiectasis is an irreversible dilation of the airways, more commonly seen in dogs than cats. Bronchiectasis typically occurs as a result of chronic airway inflammation. Dogs with ciliary dyskinesia are at risk due to their impaired mucociliary clearance function. The ventral distribution of the alveolar pattern in this case makes pneumonia, either an aspiration pneumonia or bronchopneumonia, the most likely radiographic diagnosis.

CASE 1.40

1 **What are your radiographic findings?** The cardiac silhouette appears too large for the thorax, too tall and too wide, and has a rounded shape. The trachea is dorsally displaced. The left atrium does not appear enlarged, as there is preservation of the caudal cardiac waist. What is striking is the lack of lung inflation on all three views. On the left lateral view, there is collapse of the terminal trachea

and mainstem bronchi. The cervical tracheal lumen has increased soft tissue opacity, extending into the thorax, indicative of a redundant tracheal membrane. The pulmonary blood vessels are not large and the lobar arteries and veins are matched. There is no increase in pulmonary opacity to indicate pulmonary edema. The patient is obese and the liver is enlarged.

2 What is your radiographic diagnosis? Poor pulmonary inflation with dynamic tracheal and mainstem bronchial collapse; possible cardiomegaly; no evidence of heart failure.

Comment: Poorly inflated lungs indicate either an upper airway obstruction, such as laryngeal paralysis or severe tracheal collapse, or restrictive lung disease. Because the lungs are not properly inflated, the heart appears relatively large (increased cardiothoracic ratio). Determining if it is truly large is difficult in this case, but since the left atrium does not appear large, this is evidence that there is not significant left-sided cardiomegaly. Poorly inflated lungs also render interpretation of lung disease difficult at best, since the lung parenchyma will be more opaque.

In a case such as this, it is important to try and determine if the clinical presentation of coughing and wheezing is due to heart disease or respiratory disease, or both.

Final diagnosis: Cardiac ultrasound showed mild mitral valve insufficiency and mild left ventricular enlargement. However, the patient was not in heart failure. The coughing and wheezing were attributed to tracheal membrane redundancy, with obesity contributing to poor diaphragmatic excursion and subsequent poor lung inflation ('Pickwickian' syndrome).

CASE 1.41

1 What are your radiographic findings? A large, well-defined gas opacity, with rounded margins, is present extending from the left mid-thorax to the left cranial abdomen, across the diaphragm. This structure is deviating the trachea, pulmonary structures, and cardiac silhouette primarily to the right. A mild increase in soft tissue opacity is present in the lungs, most consistent with poor aeration secondary to compression. The liver can be identified in the cranial abdomen; however, the stomach is not visualized.

2 What is your radiographic diagnosis? Diaphragmatic herniation of the stomach.

3 Is additional imaging needed? Positional radiography, oral barium contrast, peritoneography (with iodinated contrast), or ultrasound may be helpful to confirm a case of diaphragmatic herniation, if survey radiographs do not provide a clear diagnosis. In this case, the diagnosis is easier because the stomach is filled with gas.

CASE 1.42

1 What are your radiographic findings? A large soft tissue opacity, with multiple linear gas lucencies, is present in the caudal mediastinum, dorsal to the caudal vena cava and overlying the diaphragm. This soft tissue opacity is in the region of the esophagus and has an almost 'textile' appearance. The remainder of the thorax is within normal limits.

2 What is your radiographic diagnosis? Esophageal foreign body.

3 Is additional imaging needed? The location of this lesion is most consistent with the esophagus and the appearance of the lesion makes foreign material the most likely differential diagnosis. However, if unsure, an esophagram using barium or iodinated contrast could be performed to determine the location of the lesion relative to the esophagus.

Final diagnosis: Esophageal obstruction secondary to a rawhide bone foreign body.

CASE 1.43

1 What are your radiographic findings? The esophagus is focally dilated with gas in the cranial thorax, causing ventral deviation of the trachea. On the ventrodorsal view, the trachea is also deviated to the left focally at the level of T3. The cardiac silhouette and pulmonary parenchyma are within normal limits, without evidence of aspiration pneumonia. Incidentally, the 13th thoracic vertebral body is wedge-shaped and causing mild caudal thoracic kyphosis, which is not uncommon for the breed.

2 What is your radiographic diagnosis? Focal cranial thoracic megaesophagus. The primary differential diagnosis in this case is a vascular ring anomaly.

3 Is additional imaging needed? Not necessary in this case. An esophagram could be performed to confirm the narrowing of the esophagus if the radiographic findings are not adequate for making the diagnosis. Also, a CT examination could be performed to better define and assess the vascular ring anomaly, if indicated.

Final diagnosis: Persistent right aortic arch.

CASE 1.44

1 What are your radiographic findings? The lung lobes are easily identified, being of soft tissue opacity and retracted from the parietal pleura. The caudal and accessory lung lobes lungs have lost some of their volume (partial atelectasis) while the cranial lobes are almost fully inflated (based on the dorsoventral view). The right caudal lung is the most consolidated, with air bronchograms noted (alveolar pattern). Although nearly the same size as the right caudal lung lobe, the left caudal lung lobe it is not as opaque. Gas is present within the pleural space. The cardiac silhouette is deviated from the sternum and its margin partially silhouetted by the lung pathology. Rib fractures are not present.

2 What is your radiographic diagnosis? Moderate bilateral pneumothorax; pulmonary contusion worse in the right caudal lung.

Comment: The consolidation of the right caudal lung lobe is presumed secondary to pulmonary hemorrhage or contusion. Its opacity is greater than expected for simple partial atelectasis (atelectasis is defined as volume loss and can be partial, as in this case, or complete). It should be apparent that any loss of lung volume will create a more opaque lung. By comparing the right and left caudal lung lobes, the effect of volume loss on lung opacity (left) versus that created by hemorrhage can be seen.

Separation of the heart from the sternum is a radiographic sign of pneumothorax, created by loss of support of the heart by retracted lung lobes. This sign alone should not be used as the only sign by which to diagnose pneumothorax, as in some patients there is notable retraction due to thoracic conformation and large amounts of pericardial fat. This appearance is usually more pronounced on the left lateral view of the canine thorax. Here is an instance where it is important to note the difference between fat opacity and air, one of the principles of radiographic interpretation. Failure to do so may result in a misdiagnosis of pneumothorax and incorrect therapy (i.e. the contraindicated placement of a chest tube to evacuate the nonexistent pneumothorax!).

CASE 1.45

1 What are your radiographic findings? There are two thin-walled, air-filled bullae within the right pulmonary parenchyma, visualized on both the lateral and ventrodorsal views. The largest, approximately 2.8 cm in diameter, is present in the 3rd to 4th intercostal spaces, likely within the right cranial lung lobe. The smaller bulla, approximately 2.1 cm in diameter, is present in the 7th intercostal space and likely within the right caudal lung lobe. The cardiac silhouette and pulmonary vasculature are within normal limits. Incidentally, there is mild smooth ventral spondylosis at T9/10.
2 What is your radiographic diagnosis? Two right-sided pulmonary bullae.

Comment: Pulmonary bullae can develop secondary to congenital emphysema or trauma or secondary to destruction of lung parenchyma. Often, dogs with pulmonary bullae are asymptomatic unless a bulla ruptures and creates a pneumothorax.

CASE 1.46

1 What are your radiographic findings? There is a marked amount of gas opacity dissecting throughout the subcutaneous tissues of the caudal cervical region, forelimbs, thorax, and cranial abdomen. Gas is also present in the mediastinum, highlighting the brachycephalic truck, left subclavian, trachea, and aorta. The cardiac silhouette, pulmonary vasculature, and pulmonary parenchyma are within normal limits, with no evidence of a pneumothorax. No fractures are identified in the surrounding musculoskeletal structures.

2 **What is your radiographic diagnosis?** Marked subcutaneous emphysema and pneumomediastinum. Given the severity of the subcutaneous emphysema and pneumomediastinum, damage to the trachea is the most likely differential diagnosis.

Final diagnosis: Tracheal tear.

CASE 1.47

1 **What are your radiographic findings?** The cardiac silhouette is mildly enlarged, with rounding of the right heart on the dorsoventral view. Also on the dorsoventral view, there is a focal bulge in the cardiac silhouette at 1–2 o'clock, in the region of the main pulmonary artery. The caudal pulmonary arteries, most prominent on the right, are markedly enlarged and tortuous. A mild increase in soft tissue opacity is present in the caudodorsal lungs. The lateral undulation of the thoracic wall is typical for the breed. No additional abnormalities are identified.

2 **What is your radiographic diagnosis?** Marked caudal pulmonary arterial enlargement, mild right heart enlargement with a main pulmonary artery bulge and mild caudodorsal interstitial pulmonary pattern. These signs are most consistent with pulmonary hypertension. Pulmonary hypertension can develop secondary to heartworm disease, left-sided heart disease, pulmonary disease, or can be idiopathic.

Final diagnosis: This patient was positive for heartworms.

CASE 1.48

1 **What are your radiographic findings?** A marked increase in soft tissue opacity, with rounded margins, is present cranial to the cardiac silhouette on the lateral view, with widening of the cranial mediastinum on the dorsoventral view. The cardiovascular structures and pulmonary parenchyma are within normal limits.

2 **What is your radiographic diagnosis?** Cranial mediastinal mass. The most likely differential diagnoses include lymphadenopathy, thymoma, mediastinal abscess, or mediastinal cyst.

3 **Is additional imaging needed?** Ultrasound or computed tomography could be used to further evaluate the mass and help obtain a fine needle aspirate for cytology.

Final diagnosis: Lymphosarcoma.

CASE 1.49

1 **What are your radiographic findings?** A large, fairly well-defined, soft tissue opaque mass is present within the left caudodorsal lung. Multiple, variably sized soft tissue opaque nodules are present diffusely throughout the remainder of the lung.

The cardiovascular structures are within normal limits. The caudal margins of the liver are mildly rounded and extend caudal to the costochondral junction, suggestive of hepatic enlargement.

2 What is your radiographic diagnosis? Left caudodorsal pulmonary mass with multiple pulmonary nodules. The primary differential diagnosis is neoplasia, most likely primary pulmonary neoplasia with metastatic disease. A granulomatous pneumonia can also cause pulmonary nodules, but is felt less likely given the size of the pulmonary mass.

Final diagnosis: Bronchogenic carcinoma with metastasis.

CASE 1.50

1 What are your radiographic findings? A large, well-defined soft tissue opaque mass, with rounded margins, is present in the caudodorsal thorax, causing ventral displacement of the caudal vena cava. On the ventrodorsal view, the mass is in the region of the caudal mediastinum. Cranial to this mass, there is a moderate amount of gas within the esophagus, highlighting the caudal dorsal tracheal wall ('tracheal stripe sign'). The cardiovascular structures are within normal limits. The pulmonary parenchyma is unremarkable.

2 What is your radiographic diagnosis? Large caudal mediastinal mass. Differential diagnoses include paraesophageal abscess, esophageal neoplasia (possibly secondary to *Spirocirca lupi*), mediastinal cyst, or granuloma. Additionally, although this mass is in the region of the caudal mediastinum, an accessory lung lobe mass cannot be ruled out.

3 Is additional imaging needed? An esophagram can be obtained to help determine the relationship of the esophagus to the mass. Additionally, a thoracic computed tomography examination could also be helpful in determining what structures are related to the mass and if the mass is solid or fluid-filled.

Final diagnosis: Paraesophageal cyst.

CASE 2.1 A 6-year-old male German Shepherd Dog with a 4-day history of vomiting, anorexia, and straining to defecate. You obtain these abdominal radiographs: **Figs. 2.1a, b,** right lateral projections; **Fig. 2.1c,** ventrodorsal projection.

1 What are your radiographic findings?
2 What is your radiographic diagnosis?
3 Is additional imaging needed?

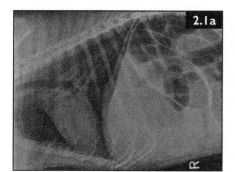
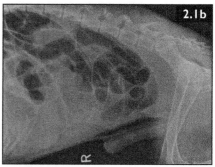

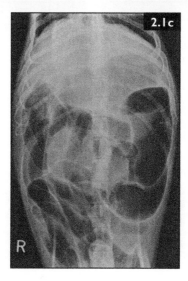

CASE 2.2 A 7-year-old female Eskimo dog with blood found under her tail. You obtain these abdominal radiographs: **Fig. 2.2a**, left lateral projection; **Fig. 2.2b**, ventrodorsal projection.

1 What are your radiographic findings?
2 What is your radiographic diagnosis?
3 Is additional imaging needed?

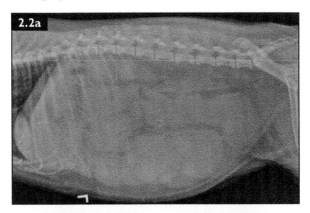

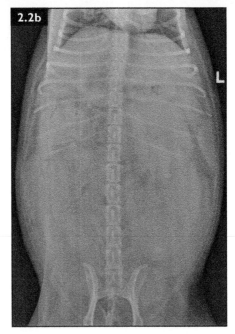

CASE 2.3 A 9-year-old spayed female German Shepherd Dog with a history of 3 months of diarrhea. You obtain these abdominal radiographs: **Fig. 2.3a**, right lateral projection; **Fig. 2.3b**, ventrodorsal projection.

1 What are your radiographic findings?
2 What is your radiographic diagnosis?
3 Is additional imaging needed?

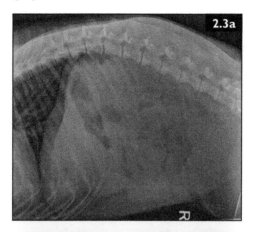

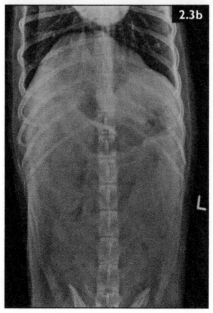

CASE 2.4 A 5-year-old spayed female Labrador Retriever with a history of lethargy and anorexia. She may have eaten some carpet 2 days ago. You obtain these abdominal radiographs: **Fig. 2.4a**, right lateral projection; **Figs. 2.4b, c**, ventrodorsal projections.

1 What are your radiographic findings?
2 What is your radiographic diagnosis?
3 Is additional imaging needed?

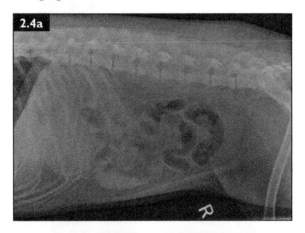

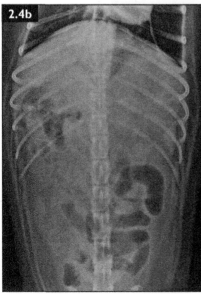

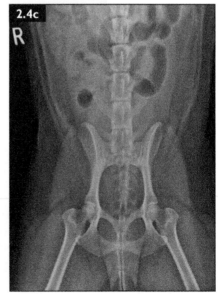

CASE 2.5 A 3-year old neutered male domestic shorthair cat found with bite wounds on right hindlimb. You obtain these abdominal radiographs: **Fig. 2.5a,** right lateral projection; **Fig. 2.5b,** ventrodorsal projection.

1 What are your radiographic findings?
2 What is your radiographic diagnosis?
3 Is additional imaging needed?

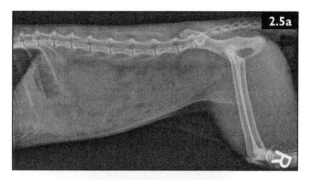

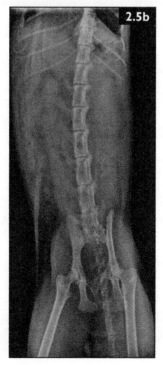

CASE 2.6 A 10-year-old spayed female mixed breed canine with chronic regurgitation and vomiting. You obtain these abdominal radiographs: **Fig. 2.6a**, right lateral projection; **Fig. 2.6b**, ventrodorsal projection.

1 What are your radiographic findings?
2 What is your radiographic diagnosis?
3 Is additional imaging needed?

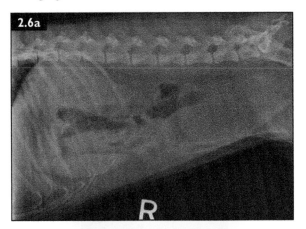

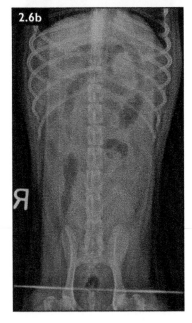

CASE 2.7 An 11-year-old male Akita, acutely lethargic and retching. You obtain these abdominal radiographs: **Fig. 2.7a**, right lateral projection; **Fig. 2.7b**, ventrodorsal projection.

1 What are your radiographic findings?
2 What is your radiographic diagnosis?

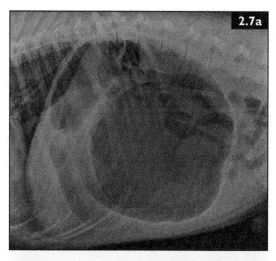

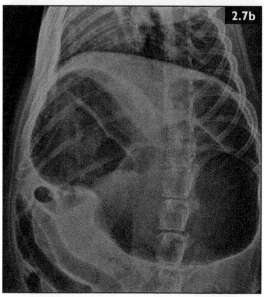

CASE 2.8 An 11-year-old spayed female Golden Retriever with a 1-day duration of lethargy and vomiting. You obtain these abdominal radiographs: **Fig. 2.8a**, left lateral projection; **Fig. 2.8b**, ventrodorsal projection.

1 What are your radiographic findings?
2 What is your radiographic diagnosis?
3 Is additional imaging needed?

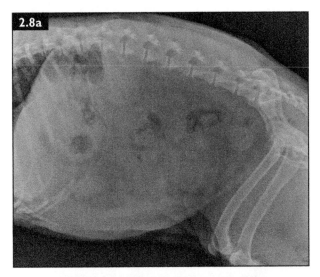

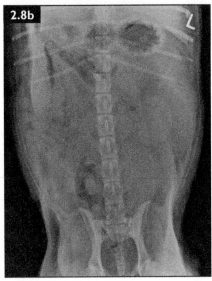

CASE 2.9 A 10-year-old male Beagle with lethargy and anorexia. You obtain this abdominal radiograph: **Fig. 2.9a**, right lateral projection.

1 What are your radiographic findings?
2 What is your radiographic diagnosis?
3 Is additional imaging needed?

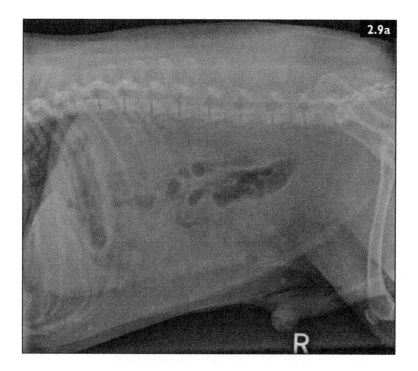

CASE 2.10 A 7-year-old spayed female mixed breed canine with stranguria and hematuria. You obtain these abdominal radiographs: **Fig. 2.10a**, right lateral projection; **Fig. 2.10b**, ventrodorsal projection.

1 What are your radiographic findings?
2 What is your radiographic diagnosis?
3 Are additional radiographic views needed?

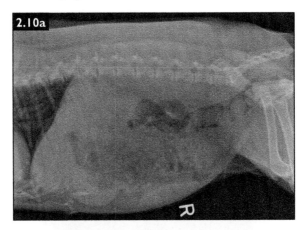

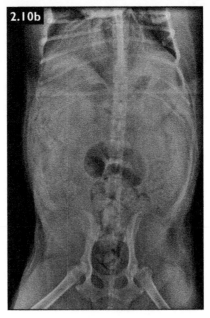

CASE 2.11 An 18-year-old spayed female Yorkshire Terrier with vomiting, diarrhea, anorexia, and a fever. You obtain these abdominal radiographs: **Fig. 2.11a,** right lateral projection; **Fig. 2.11b,** ventrodorsal projection.

1 What are your radiographic findings?
2 What is your radiographic diagnosis?
3 Is additional imaging needed?

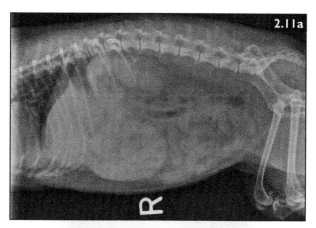

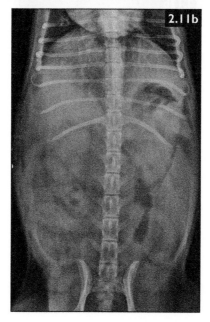

CASE 2.12 A 2-year-old male domestic shorthair cat with acute vomiting and a tense abdomen. You obtain these abdominal radiographs: **Fig. 2.12a**, right lateral projection; **Fig. 2.12b**, ventrodorsal view.

1 What are your radiographic findings?
2 What is your radiographic diagnosis?
3 Is additional imaging needed?

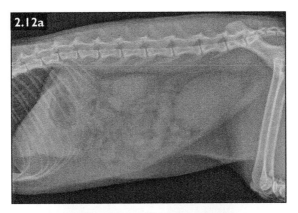

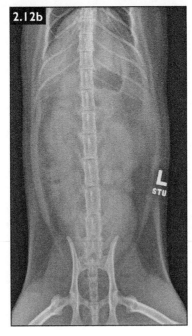

CASE 2.13 An 11-year-old neutered male domestic shorthair cat with acute lethargy, anorexia and abdominal discomfort. You obtain these abdominal radiographs: Fig. 2.13a, right lateral projection; Fig. 2.13b, ventrodorsal projection.

1 What are your radiographic findings?
2 What is your radiographic diagnosis?
3 Is additional imaging needed?

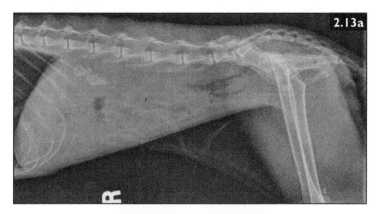

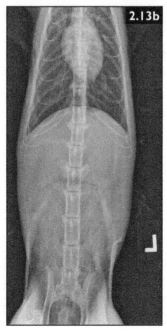

CASE 2.14 A 5-year-old female Border Collie with acute abdominal distension. You obtain these abdominal radiographs: **Fig. 2.14a**, right lateral projection; **Fig. 2.14b**, ventrodorsal projection.

1 What are your radiographic findings?
2 What is your radiographic diagnosis?

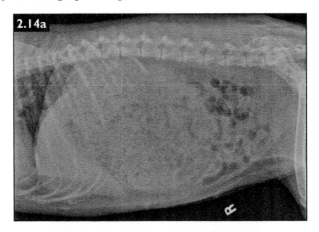

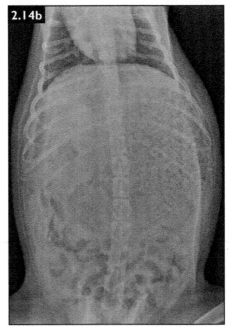

CASE 2.15 A 10-year-old spayed female Beagle with a distended abdomen. You obtain these abdominal radiographs: **Fig. 2.15a**, left lateral projection; **Figs. 2.15b, c**, ventrodorsal projections.

1 What are your radiographic findings?
2 What is your radiographic diagnosis?
3 Are additional radiographic views needed?

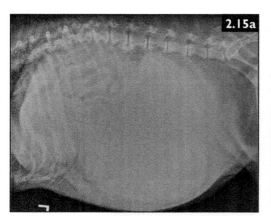
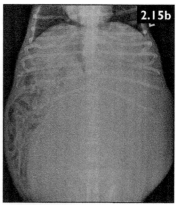

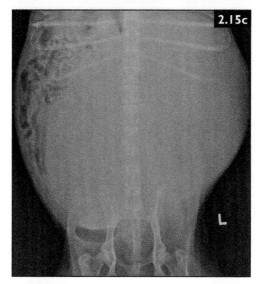

CASE 2.16 A 9-year-old male Labrador Retriever with severe ventral edema and pyoderma, hindlimb swelling, and straining when urinating/defecating. You obtain these abdominal radiographs: **Figs. 2.16a, b**, left lateral projections; **Figs. 2.16c, d**, ventrodorsal projections.

1 What are your radiographic findings?
2 What is your radiographic diagnosis?
3 Is additional imaging needed?

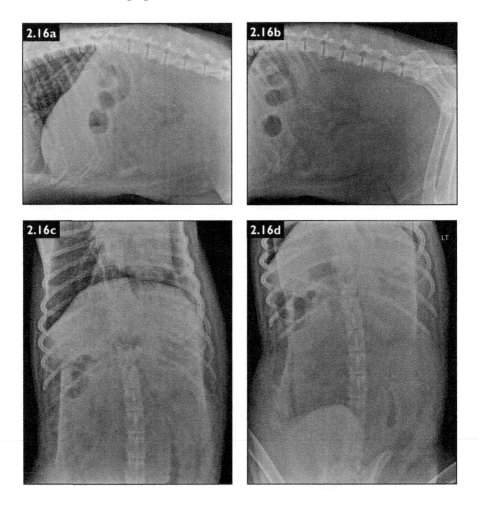

CASE 2.17 A 5-year-old female canine presented for dystocia and a brown exudate was visualized around the vulva. You obtain these abdominal radiographs: Fig. 2.17a, left lateral projection; Fig. 2.17b, ventrodorsal projection.

1 What are your radiographic findings?
2 What is your radiographic diagnosis?
3 Is additional imaging needed?

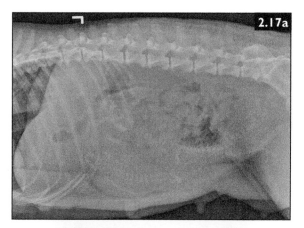

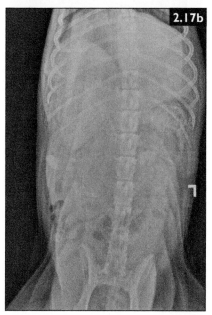

CASE 2.18 A 10-year-old spayed female domestic shorthair cat with anorexia. The owner reports that the cat is vocalizing more at home. You obtain these abdominal radiographs: **Fig. 2.18a**, left lateral projection; **Fig. 2.18b**, ventrodorsal projection.

1 What are your radiographic findings?
2 What is your radiographic diagnosis?
3 Is additional imaging needed?

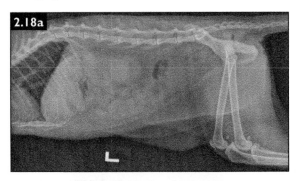

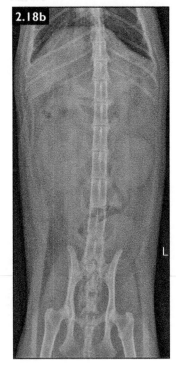

CASE 2.19 An 11-year-old neutered male Rat Terrier with a history of constipation and elevated liver enzymes on a blood chemistry panel. You obtain these abdominal radiographs: **Fig. 2.19a**, left lateral projection; **Fig. 2.19b**, ventrodorsal projection.

1 What are your radiographic findings?
2 What is your radiographic diagnosis?
3 Is additional imaging needed?

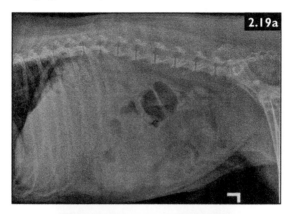

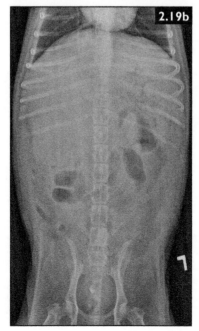

CASE 2.20 A 13-year-old neutered male Jack Russell Terrier with a history of vomiting. An abdominal exploratory was performed the previous day and no abnormalities of the gastrointestinal tract identified. At presentation, the abdomen was distended and tense on palpation. Additionally, the patient has a history of a previous mass removal (mast cell tumor) dorsal to the lumbar vertebral bodies. You obtain these abdominal radiographs: **Fig. 2.20a**, left lateral projection; **Fig. 2.20b**, ventrodorsal projection.

1 What are your radiographic findings?
2 What is your radiographic diagnosis?
3 Is additional imaging needed?

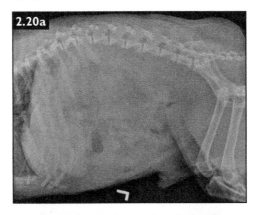

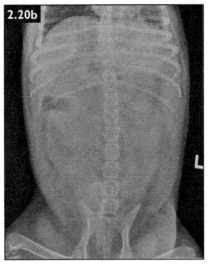

CASE 2.21 A 6-year-old spayed female Labrador Retriever with a history of lethargy and abdominal discomfort. You obtain these abdominal radiographs: Fig. 2.21a, right lateral projection; 2.21b, c, ventrodorsal projections.

1 What are your radiographic findings?
2 What is your radiographic diagnosis?
3 Is additional imaging needed?

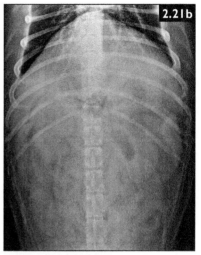

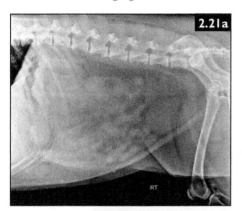

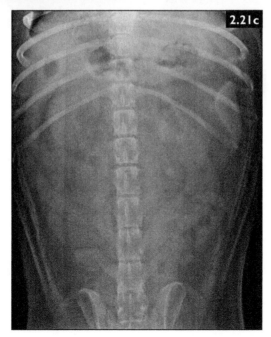

CASE 2.22 A 6-year-old spayed female Boxer with a 1-week history of lethargy, inappetence, and vomiting blood. You obtain these abdominal radiographs: **Figs. 2.22a, b,** left lateral projections; **Figs. 2.22c, d,** ventrodorsal projections.

1 What are your radiographic findings?
2 What is your radiographic diagnosis?
3 Is additional imaging needed?

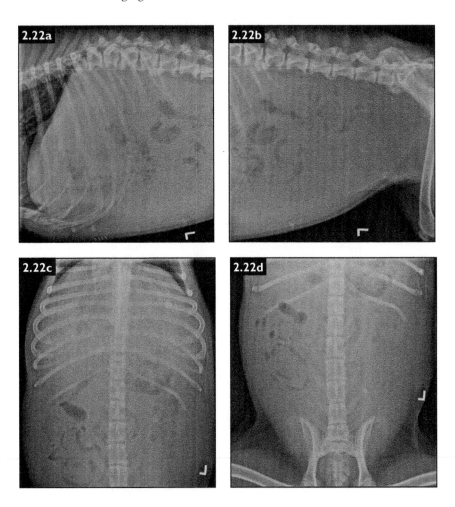

CASE 2.23 A 12-year-old neutered male Maltese with a history of hematuria and a portosystemic shunt (surgically corrected as a puppy). You obtain these abdominal radiographs: **Fig. 2.23a**, left lateral projection; **Fig. 2.23b**, ventrodorsal projection.

1 What are your radiographic findings?
2 What is your radiographic diagnosis?
3 Is additional imaging needed?

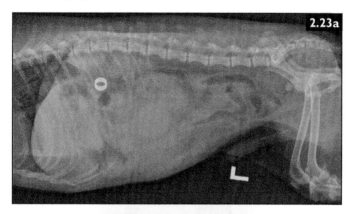

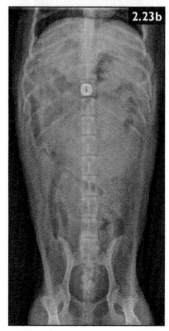

CASE 2.24 A 13-year-old neutered male domestic shorthair cat with a prior diagnosis of nasal lymphoma and vomiting after administration of chemotherapy. You obtain these abdominal radiographs: **Fig. 2.24a**, left lateral projection; **Fig. 2.24b**, ventrodorsal projection.

1 What are your radiographic findings?
2 What is your radiographic diagnosis?
3 Is additional imaging needed?

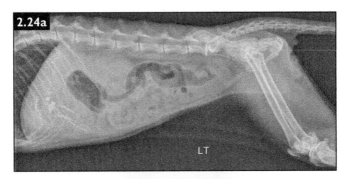

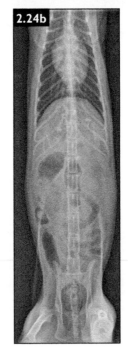

CASE 2.25 A 2-year-old neutered male mixed breed dog with a 2-week history of vomiting and diarrhea. You obtain these abdominal radiographs: **Fig. 2.25a**, left lateral projection; **Fig. 2.25b**, ventrodorsal projection.

1 What are your radiographic findings?
2 What is your radiographic diagnosis?
3 Is additional imaging needed?

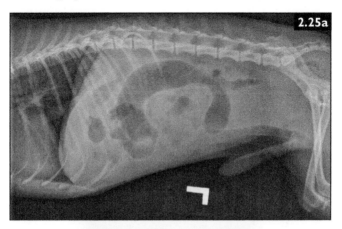

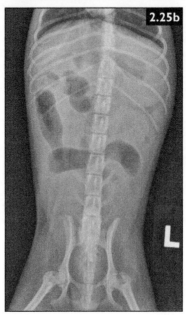

CASE 2.26 Old dog with hematuria. An intravenous pyelogram (IVP, also known as excretory urogram [EU]) was performed and a single lateral image is provided (**Fig. 2.26a**). An ultrasound image of the urinary bladder was also obtained (**Fig. 2.26b**).

1 What are your imaging findings?
2 What is your imaging diagnosis?

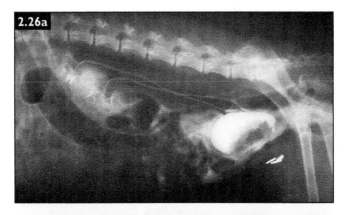

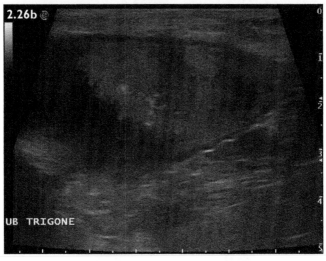

CASE 2.27 A 10-year-old neutered male domestic shorthair cat with a several months history of intermittent vomiting and diarrhea. You obtain these abdominal radiographs: **Fig. 2.27a**, left lateral projection; **Fig. 2.27b**, ventrodorsal projection.

1 What are your radiographic findings?
2 What is your radiographic diagnosis?
3 Is additional imaging needed?

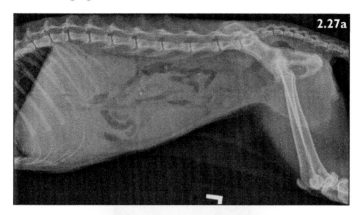

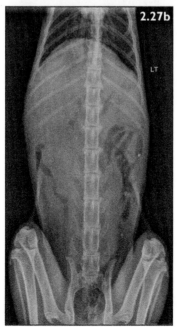

CASE 2.28 A 3-year-old spayed female Manx cat who has not defecated in 3 days. You obtain these abdominal radiographs: **Fig. 2.28a**, left lateral projection; **Fig. 2.28b**, ventrodorsal projection.

1 What are your radiographic findings?
2 What is your radiographic diagnosis?
3 Is additional imaging needed?

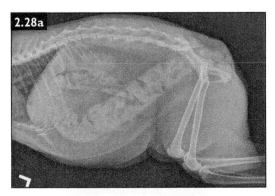

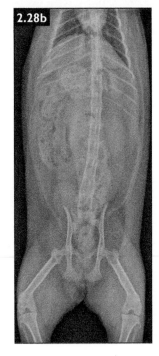

CASE 2.29 A 9-year-old spayed female English Setter with a 10-day history of lethargy and fever, and elevated liver enzymes on a serum chemistry. You obtain these abdominal radiographs: **Figs. 2.29a, b**, left lateral projections; **Figs. 2.29c, d**, ventrodorsal projections.

1 What are your radiographic findings?
2 What is your radiographic diagnosis?
3 Is additional imaging needed?

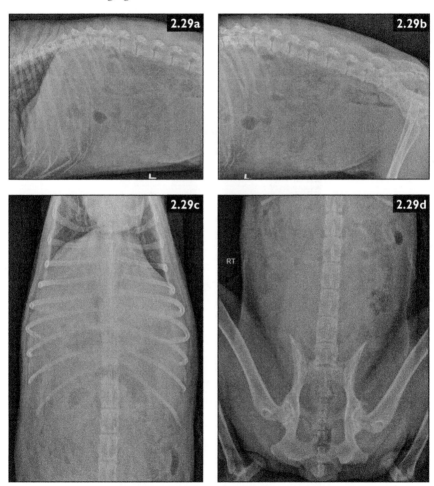

CASE 2.30 A 2-year-old female domestic shorthair cat with a history of lethargy, inappetence, and abdominal pain. You obtain these abdominal radiographs: **Fig. 2.30a**, left lateral projection; **Fig. 2.30b**, ventrodorsal projection.

1 What are your radiographic findings?
2 What is your radiographic diagnosis?

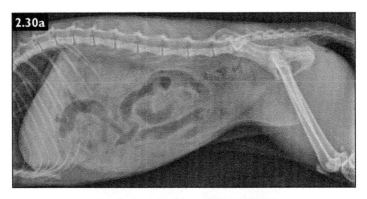

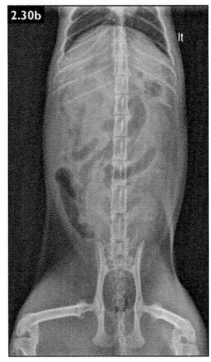

CASE 2.31 A 5-year-old neutered male Siamese cat with lethargy and weight loss. You obtain these abdominal radiographs: **Fig. 2.31a**, left lateral projection; **Fig. 2.31b**, ventrodorsal projection.

1 What are your radiographic findings?
2 What is your radiographic diagnosis?
3 Is additional imaging needed?

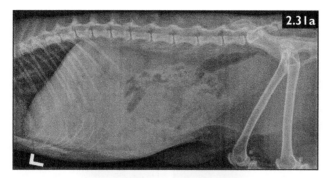

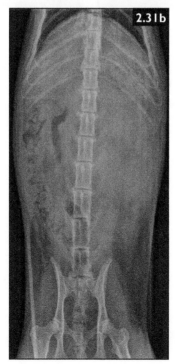

CASE 2.32 A 4-year-old male Doberman Pinscher with a 2-week history of hematuria. You obtain these abdominal radiographs: **Figs. 2.32a, b**, left lateral projections; **Figs. 2.32c, d**, ventrodorsal projections.

1 What are your radiographic findings?
2 What is your radiographic diagnosis?
3 Is additional imaging needed?

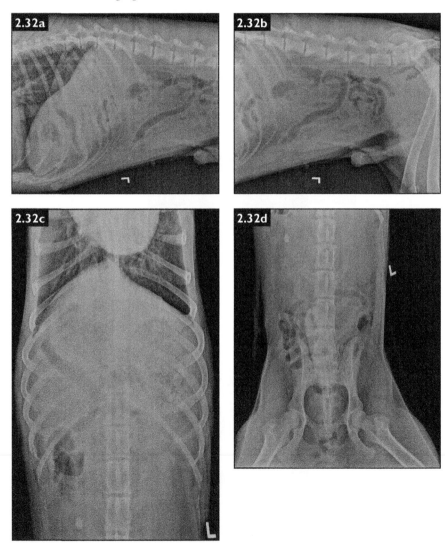

CASE 2.33 A 6-year-old spayed female Siberian Husky vomiting for the past 24 hours. You obtain these abdominal radiographs: **Fig. 2.33a**, left lateral projection; **Fig. 2.33b**, ventrodorsal projection.

1 What are your radiographic findings?
2 What is your radiographic diagnosis?
3 Is additional imaging needed?

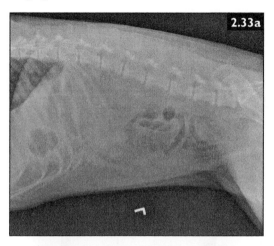

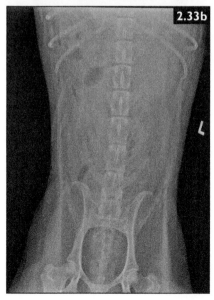

CASE 2.34 An 11-year-old spayed female Pekingese with a history of prior surgical removal of the left adrenal gland and bladder stones. You obtain these abdominal radiographs: **Fig. 2.34a**, left lateral projection; **Fig. 2.34b**, ventrodorsal projection.

1 What are your radiographic findings?
2 What is your radiographic diagnosis?
3 Is additional imaging needed?

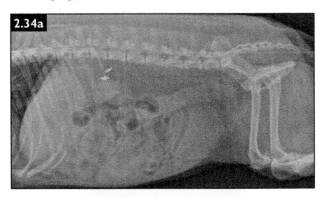

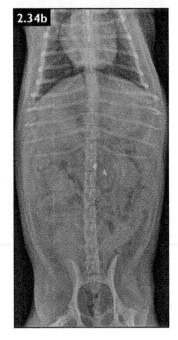

CASE 2.35 A 13-year-old spayed female cat, possibly attacked by dog 3 hours ago. You obtain these abdominal radiographs: **Fig. 2.35a**, right lateral projection; **Fig. 2.35b**, ventrodorsal projection.

1 What are your radiographic findings?
2 What is your radiographic diagnosis?
3 Is additional imaging needed?

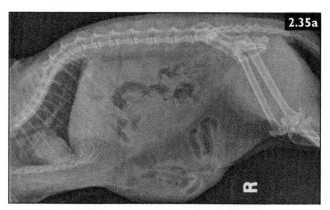

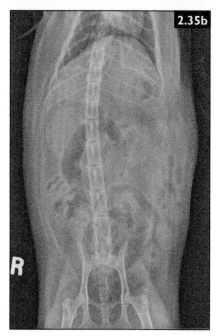

113

CASE 2.36 An 11-year-old neutered male Cocker Spaniel with inappetence, lethargy, and intermittent vomiting. You obtain these abdominal radiographs: **Fig. 2.36a**, left lateral projection; **Fig. 2.36b**, ventrodorsal projection.

1 What are your radiographic findings?
2 What is your radiographic diagnosis?
3 Is additional imaging needed?

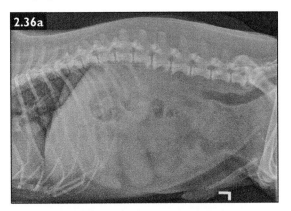

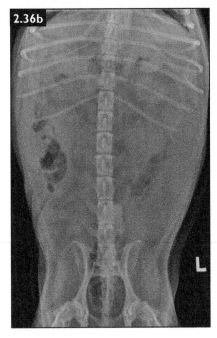

CASE 2.37 A 6-year-old neutered male Cairn Terrier with decreased appetite and a 'bloated' appearance. You obtain these abdominal radiographs: **Fig. 2.37a**, left lateral projection; **Fig. 2.37b**, ventrodorsal projection.

1 What are your radiographic findings?
2 What is your radiographic diagnosis?
3 Is additional imaging needed?

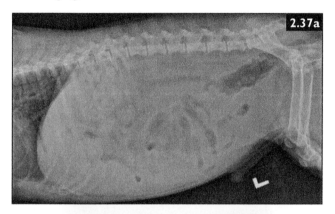

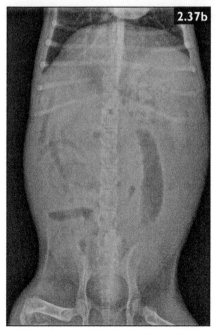

CASE 2.38 A 6-year-old spayed female Miniature Schnauzer with a history of vomiting and an enlarged abdomen. You obtain these abdominal radiographs: **Fig. 2.38a**, left lateral projection; **Fig. 2.38b**, ventrodorsal projection.

1 What are your radiographic findings?
2 What is your radiographic diagnosis?
3 Is additional imaging needed?

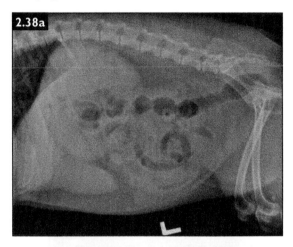

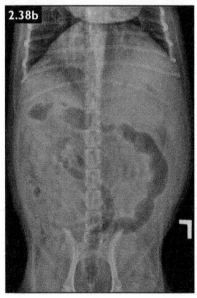

CASE 2.39 A 16-year-old Dachshund with intermittent vomiting, occasionally with blood. You obtain these radiographs following oral administration of barium contrast: **Fig. 2.39a**, left lateral projection; **Fig. 2.39b**, ventrodorsal projection.

1 What are your radiographic findings?
2 What is your radiographic diagnosis?
3 Are additional radiograph views needed?

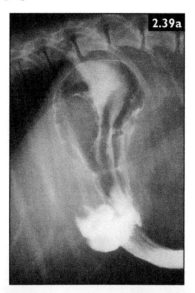

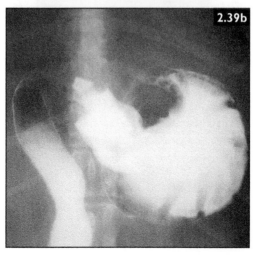

CASE 2.40 A 12-year-old neutered male Labrador Retriever with difficulty urinating and dribbling urine. You obtain these abdominal radiographs: **Fig. 2.40a**, left lateral projection of the caudal abdomen; **Fig. 2.40b**, left lateral projection of the caudal abdomen with legs pulled forward; **Fig. 2.40c**, ventrodorsal projection of the caudal abdomen.

1 What are your radiographic findings?
2 What is your radiographic diagnosis?
3 Is additional imaging needed?

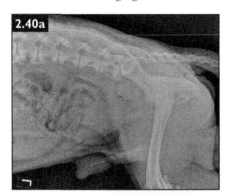

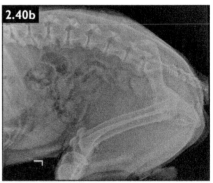

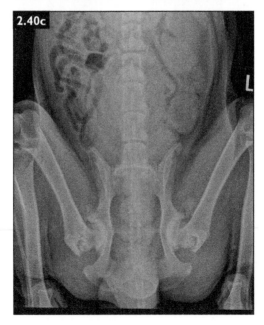

CASE 2.41 A 16-year-old neutered male Toy Poodle with lethargy, inappetence, and hypoglycemia. You obtain these abdominal radiographs: **Fig. 2.41a**, left lateral projection; **Fig. 2.41b**, ventrodorsal projection.

1 What are your radiographic findings?
2 What is your radiographic diagnosis?
3 Is additional imaging needed?

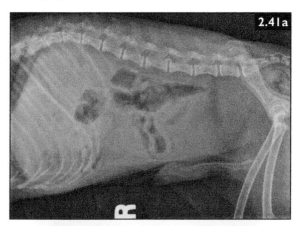

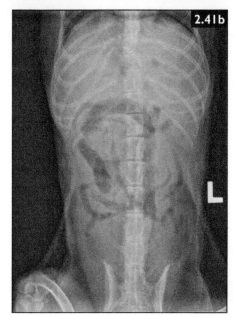

CASE 2.42 A 5-year-old neutered male Golden Retriever with severe vomiting and nausea. You obtain these abdominal radiographs: **Fig. 2.42a,** ventrodorsal projection of the stomach and duodenum made 30 minutes after barium administration; **Fig. 2.42b,** close-up ventrodorsal view of the proximal duodenum made 2 hours later.

1 What are your radiographic findings?
2 What is your radiographic diagnosis?

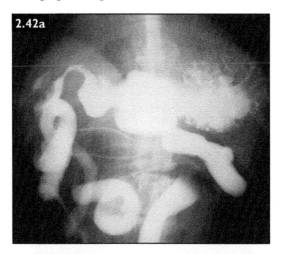

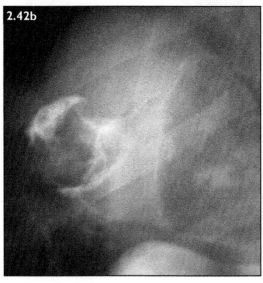

CASE 2.43 An 8-year-old male Dachshund with a history of perineal swelling. On physical examination, a perineal hernia was present. You obtain these abdominal radiographs: **Fig. 2.43a**, ventrodorsal projection; **Fig. 2.43b**, ventrodorsal projection.

1 What are your radiographic findings?
2 What is your radiographic diagnosis?
3 Is additional imaging needed?

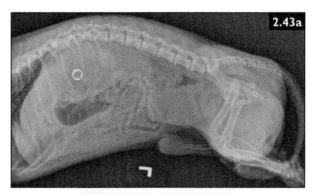

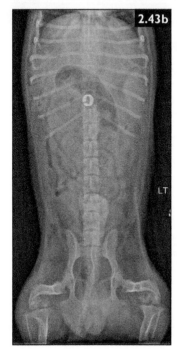

CASE 2.44 An 8-year-old spayed female Pomeranian with a 2-day history of vomiting and diarrhea. You obtain these abdominal radiographs: **Fig. 2.44a**, right lateral projection; **Fig. 2.44b**, ventrodorsal projection.

1 What are your radiographic findings?
2 What is your radiographic diagnosis?
3 Is additional imaging needed?

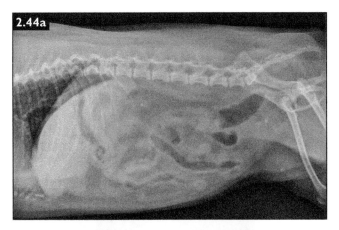

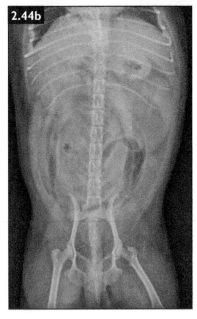

CASE 2.45 An older cat with renal failure. You obtain these abdominal radiographs: **Fig. 2.45a**, lateral projection; **Fig. 2.45b**, ventrodorsal projection.

1 What are your radiographic findings?
2 What is your radiographic diagnosis?
3 Is additional imaging needed?

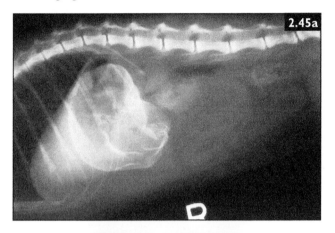

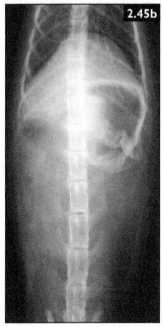

CASE 2.1

1 What are your radiographic findings? The loops of small intestine are diffusely distended with gas and fluid opacities. The largest gas distended bowel likely represents the colon. Note that the descending colon is not seen at the pelvic inlet. The remainder of the abdominal structures are within normal limits. The cardiac silhouette is markedly reduced in size, as seen on the cranial right lateral view.

2 What is your radiographic diagnosis? Severe small and large intestinal dilation. The severity of the findings suggest a mesenteric root torsion, including a colonic torsion, or a distal small intestinal obstruction (e.g. foreign body).

3 Is additional imaging needed? No.

Comment: Given the severity of the radiographic findings and the protracted and severe clinical history and signs, surgical exploration is indicated following rehydration and stabilization of the patient.

CASE 2.2

1 What are your radiographic findings? A large, smoothly marginated tubular soft tissue opaque structure is present occupying the majority of the caudal abdomen. This structure is causing displacement of the adjacent abdominal viscera, including dorsal displacement of the small bowel and ventral displacement of the apex of the urinary bladder. The loops of small bowel are normal in size. The urinary bladder is moderately distended with urine. The abdominal serosal detail is within normal limits. The surrounding musculoskeletal structures are within normal limits.

2 What is your radiographic diagnosis? Enlarged soft tissue, tubular caudal abdominal structure, most consistent with an enlarged uterus. Differential diagnoses for an enlarged uterus include mucometra, hydrometra, or pyometra.

3 Is additional imaging needed? Ultrasound can be used to confirm the dilated tubular structure is actually uterus, although this is not needed in many cases. An example of the fluid distended uterus in this case is shown (**Fig. 2.2c**).

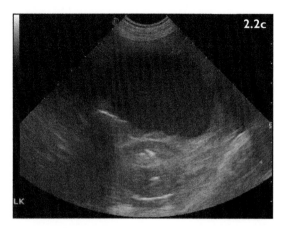

125

Comment: The uterine body, located between the colon and urinary bladder, could not be identified on the radiographs due to its small size. Commonly, in cases of severely fluid-filled uterine horns, the uterine body will actually be small as fluid accumulates in the more gravitationally dependent horns.

Final diagnosis: Pyometra.

CASE 2.3

1 What are your radiographic findings? The serosal detail within the mid-abdomen on the lateral view and primarily on the right on the ventrodorsal view is decreased. However, the detail within the cranioventral abdomen, between the liver and falciform fat, is maintained. Some loops of small intestine are mildly dilated; however, the dimensions of the loops are difficult to appreciate due to the loss of serosal detail. Note the left kidney is easily identified on the ventrodorsal view due to its retroperitoneal location and normal retroperitoneal detail.

2 What is your radiographic diagnosis? Decreased abdominal serosal detail. Differential diagnoses include peritoneal effusion, mesenteric inflammation, or peritoneal masses (i.e. carcinomatosis). Additional causes of decreased serosal detail include young age (lack of fat or fat with increased water content) or being underweight (lack of fat to provide contrast to the soft tissue organs); however, these can be excluded as differentials in this specific patient.

3 Is additional imaging needed? An abdominal ultrasound could be considered for further assessment of conformation of the radiographic findings.

Final diagnosis: Carcinomatosis. Multiple abdominal masses were found at exploratory surgery, which were histopathologically determined to be carcinoma.

CASE 2.4

1 What are your radiographic findings? Multiple small intestinal loops in the cranial and mid-abdomen are distended. The small bowel loops in the cranial abdomen contain primarily granular soft tissue opacity, while the more caudal loops contain primarily gas opacity. Additionally, multiple loops also appear folded with an undulating contour, most consistent with plication. No fecal material is evident in the colon. The abdominal serosal detail is within normal limits.

2 What is your radiographic diagnosis? Small intestinal linear foreign body obstruction.

3 Is additional imaging needed? If survey radiographs are inconclusive, an ultrasound or upper gastrointestinal contrast study, using barium, may be indicated.

Comment: Linear foreign bodies often cause the small bowel to have an abnormal gas pattern and contour. In patients with linear foreign bodies, numerous small gas bubbles, which may be crescent-shaped, are evident. Additionally, the loops of bowel become pleated or plicated in appearance due to hyperperistalsis.

Final diagnosis: Linear foreign body (carpet).

CASE 2.5

1 What are your radiographic findings? Both kidneys are enlarged, primarily too wide, with normal margination. The urinary bladder is moderately distended. Urinary calculi are not visualized. The small intestines are fluid and gas filled, evenly distributed throughout the abdominal cavity, and normal in size. The stomach and colon are relatively empty. The liver is mildly enlarged, extending beyond the costal arch on the lateral view with rounded caudal margins. The spleen is normal in size, visualized along the left body wall. The patient is mildly rotated on the ventrodorsal view; however, this does not hinder interpretation.

2 What is your radiographic diagnosis? Bilateral renomegaly, mild hepatomegaly. Differential diagnoses for bilateral kidney enlargement are many and include acute nephritis, severe pyelonephritis, hydronephrosis, lymphoma, feline infectious peritonitis (FIP), or polycystic kidney disease.

3 Is additional imaging needed? An ultrasound examination would be the next diagnostic imaging test. Ultrasound can differentiate hydronephrosis and polycystic renal disease from solid parenchymal diseases such as lymphoma, FIP, and acute nephritis.

Comment: A fine needle aspirate of the kidneys would be diagnostic in cases of lymphoma, whereas tissue core biopsies may be needed to diagnosis FIP and acute nephritis. Blood work (complete blood count and serum chemistry) and a urinalysis should be performed. FeLV/FIV testing could also be performed, and in this case was negative.

CASE 2.6

1 What are your radiographic findings? The duodenum is gas filled on both views and mildly enlarged. The remaining small intestine is strikingly different in its appearance, being empty and much smaller in size. The remainder of the examination is normal, with excellent abdominal detail outlining the stomach and remaining small intestine, liver, spleen, and urinary bladder.

2 What is your radiographic diagnosis? Gas-dilated duodenum. Differential diagnoses include inflammation, neoplasia, or radiolucent foreign material. Duodenitis secondary to pancreatitis is another consideration, although the excellent abdominal detail and normal position of the duodenum and colon does not support pancreatitis as an etiology for the appearance of the duodenum.

3 Is additional imaging needed? Differentiating the colon from the small intestine can be difficult in some cases. In this case, the gas- and feces-filled descending colon can be followed orad on the ventrodorsal view to the transverse colon, which is clearly a separate loop of bowel from the duodenum. An upper gastrointestinal contrast study using liquid barium or ultrasound of the duodenum should be considered. You obtain the following barium contrast study images: **Figs. 2.6c, e,** right lateral projections at 5 minutes and 5 hours; **Figs. 2.6d, f,** ventrodorsal projections at 5 minutes and 5 hours, respectively.

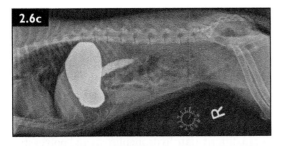

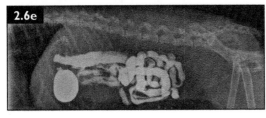

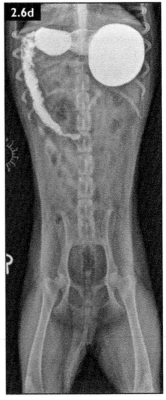

Comment: The duodenum is still dilated and is irregularly filled with barium. Irregular projections of barium are present within the wall of the duodenum, indicative of mucosal erosions and thickening. The duodenal appearance is essentially unchanged over the 5-hour period. The barium continues through the small intestine and is present in the ascending and transverse colon by 5 hours. However, the stomach still contains a large portion of the barium at 5 hours, indicative of delayed gastric emptying.

The radiographic diagnosis is infiltrative duodenal disease with markedly prolonged gastric emptying. The duodenal pathology is consistent with a severe inflammatory or infiltrative process of the duodenum. Differential diagnoses include lymphoma, fungal infection, or inflammatory bowel disease.

Final diagnosis: Lymphoma.

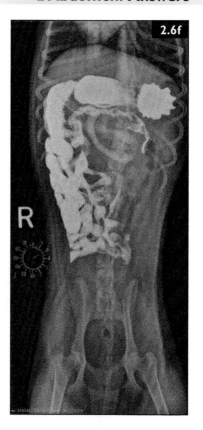

2.6f

CASE 2.7

1 What are your radiographic findings? The stomach is severely gas distended. The pylorus is displaced cranially and dorsally, creating a fold of soft tissue separating it from the gastric body ('compartmentalization'). The small intestinal loops caudal to the stomach are gas filled, although normal in size.

2 What is your radiographic diagnosis? Gastric dilatation and volvulus (GDV).

Comment: Classic radiographic features of GDV are distension of the stomach (primarily with gas), displacement of the pylorus dorsally and to the left, a soft tissue opaque fold along the gas-filled lumen (compartmentalization), caudal displacement of other structures (i.e. small bowel) from the distended stomach, and potentially splenomegaly due to disruption of normal blood supply. A right lateral view can be used alone to make this diagnosis; however, if unsure, additional views may be needed. If a 360-degree torsion is present, the stomach will still be gas dilated but fundus and pylorus will be in the normal position.

CASE 2.8

1 What are your radiographic findings? There is a decrease in abdominal serosal detail of the right cranial abdomen on the ventrodorsal view. The descending duodenum is gas filled, although within normal size limits, and displaced laterally to the right abdominal wall. The remainder of the small bowel is within normal limits. The left aspect of the transverse colon is caudally displaced and the proximal descending colon is positioned toward midline (ventrodorsal view). A partially spherical, smoothly marginated, faintly mineralized mass is present between the urinary bladder and colon, on midline, best visualized on the lateral view.

2 What is your radiographic diagnosis? Loss of right cranial abdominal serosal detail with displacement of the duodenum and colon is most consistent with pancreatitis. The caudal abdominal mass is most likely a mineralized uterine stump (incidental finding).

3 Is additional imaging needed? Abdominal ultrasound would be recommended for further evaluation of the pancreas. **Fig. 2.8c** shows an enlarged, hypoechoic left pancreatic lobe (between electronic calipers, 3.3 cm thick). The surrounding mesentery is hyperechoic, indicative of inflammation. **Fig. 2.8d** shows a very hyperemic left pancreatic lobe parenchyma as assessed by power Doppler, supportive of acute pancreatitis.

Final diagnosis: Pancreatitis and uterine stump granuloma.

Comment: Appreciation of the normal position of the colon is important in patients with clinical signs of pancreatitis. The left lobe of the pancreas is located between the greater curvature of the stomach and the transverse colon. The right pancreatic lobe is present between the descending duodenum and the ascending colon. Therefore, pancreatitis or pancreatic masses may cause a displacement of these organs.

The large partially mineralized caudal midline mass is located between the urinary bladder and the colon, making a mass of uterine origin the only reasonable differential diagnosis (there are no other anatomic structures located in this area). Since this patient has had an ovariohysterectomy, the diagnosis of a uterine stump

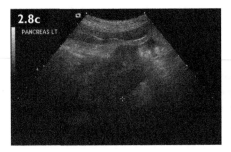

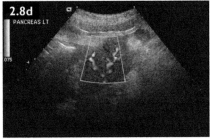

mineralizing granuloma can be made with confidence. It was clinically silent in this case, although 'stump' pyometras can be a clinical entity. Note the exquisite serosal detail surrounding the uterine stump and compare this with the appearance of the cranial abdomen on the lateral view if you are not convinced of the reduced detail.

The uterine stump granuloma, while being the most obvious radiographic abnormality, was really unimportant in this patient's clinical presentation. It can be called a 'radiographic distracter', potentially taking away from more critical assessment of the radiographic study and thus making a misdiagnosis. Ultimately, ultrasound examination was a very necessary diagnostic test in this case, as it provided the definitive diagnosis.

CASE 2.9

1 What are your radiographic findings? The prostate is enlarged with a smooth, mildly irregular contour.

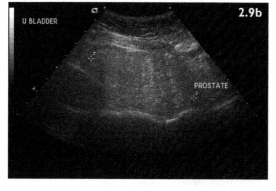

2 What is your radiographic diagnosis? Prostatomegaly. Considering the patient's intact status, benign prostatic hypertrophy is most likely. Prostatitis is also possible.

3 Is additional imaging needed? Ultrasound can be useful in further evaluating the prostate gland and obtaining an ultrasound-guided fine needle aspirate for cytology and culture. A normal prostate gland should be symmetrical in size and homogeneous in echogenicity, without cysts, mineralization, or gas. A representative ultrasound image of the prostate in this case is shown (**Fig. 2.9b**). This prostate is enlarged, although quite homogeneous.

Comment: Enlargement of the prostate is visualized as a soft tissue mass caudal to the urinary bladder and ventral to the descending colon, with potential cranial displacement of the urinary bladder and dorsal displacement of the colon. Benign prostatic hypertrophy and prostatitis are the two most common differential diagnoses for symmetric enlargement of the prostate gland. If asymmetric enlargement is present, neoplasia or prostatic or paraprostatic cysts and abscesses are the most likely causes. Mineralization of the prostate may be seen with neoplasia or chronic prostatitis. A definitive cause of the lethargy and anorexia was not identified in this case.

Final diagnosis: Benign prostatic hypertrophy.

131

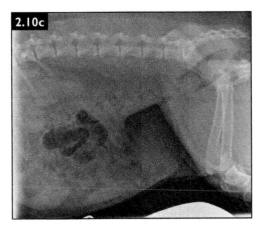

2.10c

CASE 2.10

1 What are your radiographic findings? The urinary bladder is moderately distended; however, no definitive calculi can be visualized. The colon contains a moderate amount of granular fecal material, which is superimposed with the apex of the urinary bladder on the lateral view.

2 What is your radiographic diagnosis? Given the history of this patient, urinary calculi are suspected.

3 Are additional radiographic views needed? Yes. A wooden paddle was used to compress the abdomen and move the overlying colon dorsally. The lateral image with the paddle compression is shown (**Fig. 2.10c**). Without the superimposition of the fecal material, multiple small mineral opaque calculi can now be visualized within the urinary bladder.

Comment: Calcium oxalate, struvite (phosphate), and silica calculi are radiopaque and can be distinguished from the surrounding urine on radiographs; however, other types of urinary calculi (urate and cystine) may be visualized on survey radiographs and a contrast cystogram (iodine) or ultrasound of the bladder may be needed.

Final diagnosis: Cystic calculi.

CASE 2.11

1 What are your radiographic findings? A soft tissue mass is present within the cranial abdomen. This mass is ventral to the stomach and colon on the lateral view and extends caudal to the stomach on both sides of midline on the ventrodorsal view. Multifocal, irregularly-shaped areas of gas opacity are present within the mass, best visualized on the lateral view. The caudal margins of the liver cannot be definitively identified. The splenic and kidney margins can be visualized separate from the mass. The remainder of the intra-abdominal structures are within normal limits.

2 What is your radiographic diagnosis? Cranial abdominal mass with foci of gas. The liver is the most likely origin of the mass, based on its location and difficulty in visualizing liver margins. The most likely differential diagnoses are hepatic or biliary neoplasia with necrosis or liver abscessation.

3 Is additional imaging needed? An ultrasound or computed tomography examination of the abdomen would help further evaluate this mass and determine if it is indeed originating from the liver. An ultrasound image of a liver mass with hyperechoic gas present distal to the round anechoic gallbladder, consistent with an hepatic abscess, is shown (**Fig. 2.11c**). Ultrasound-guided fine needle aspirates or biopsy of the mass could be performed for cytology/histopathology and culture.

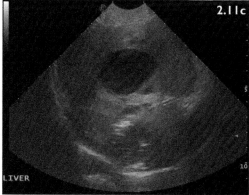

Comment: Cytology of the liver mass showed degenerative neutrophils with intra- and extracellular rod bacteria. Culture showed *Serratia* species.

Final diagnosis: Liver abscess.

CASE 2.12

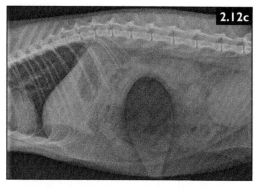

1 What are your radiographic findings? The stomach contains a small amount of gas and soft tissue opaque material/fluid. The stomach is small in size, which is typical for the history of frequent vomiting. The loops of small bowel have mildly indistinct serosal margins; however, the remainder of the abdomen has normal serosal detail. The small intestinal loops also appear bunched together on the lateral view, yet are still normal in size and contain primarily soft tissue opacity (fluid). On the ventrodorsal view, a loop of small bowel, overlying the left kidney, is undulating or plicated in appearance. The colon contains a moderate amount of granular fecal material. Incidentally, the right 13th rib is hypoplastic.

2 What is your radiographic diagnosis? Suspect small intestinal linear foreign material. The bunching of the intestines and plicated appearance of some loops make a linear foreign body the most likely differential diagnosis.

3 Is additional imaging needed? A paddle (in this case a wooden spoon) can be used to compress the abdomen and better visualize abnormal loops of bowel (**Fig. 2.12c**). The loop of bowel along the dorsal aspect of the spoon is plicated in

133

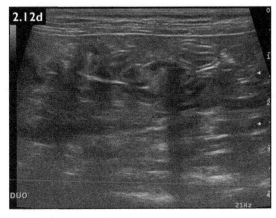

appearance, in comparison with the normal loops of bowel ventrally.

Ultrasound can also be used to confirm plication of the bowel and the foreign material can be visualized in some cases (**Fig. 2.12d**).

Final diagnosis: Linear foreign body.

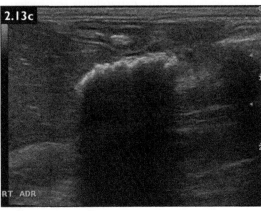

CASE 2.13

1 What are your radiographic findings? Two clearly defined structures with diffuse granular mineral foci are present in the dorsal abdomen to the left and right of midline, in the region of the adrenal glands. The kidneys cannot be seen radiographically due to lack of surrounding retroperitoneal fat. There is a moderate, diffuse decrease in abdominal serosal detail obscuring some serosal margins of organs, which is likely secondary to lack of peritoneal and retroperitoneal fat as the patient is in very thin body condition. Wet hair is superimposed with the abdomen creating wispy linear soft tissue markings.

2 What is your radiographic diagnosis? Bilateral adrenal gland mineralization.

3 Is additional imaging needed? Ultrasound can be used to further evaluate the adrenal glands. An ultrasound image of the mineralized right adrenal gland is shown (**Fig. 2.13c**). Note the strong acoustic shadow from the mineralization. Ultrasound can also be used to further investigate the cause of the clinical signs in this patient.

Comment: Adrenal gland mineralization in cats may be an incidental finding. It has been reported to be associated with muscular dystrophy. Blood work for this patient revealed renal failure.

Final diagnosis: Adrenal gland mineralization.

CASE 2.14

1 What are your radiographic findings? The stomach is markedly distended with granular soft tissue opacity, most likely food. The stomach is normal in position with the pylorus being in a right ventral position. The duodenum is mildly dilated, filled with the same material visualized within the stomach. The remainder of the small bowel contains gas and a small amount of fluid, being displaced caudally by the enlarged stomach. The colon contains formed fecal material; however, it is also displaced caudally. There is good abdominal serosal detail.

2 What is your radiographic diagnosis? Marked gastric distension, likely with food.

Comment: The owners found a large hole in the dog food bag after returning home. If the patient's abdominal distension persists or the patient develops clinical signs (i.e. vomiting), repeat radiographs of the abdomen could be considered to ensure the material/food in the stomach is emptying normally.

Final diagnosis: Food bloat.

CASE 2.15

1 What are your radiographic findings? A large soft tissue opaque mass is present occupying the majority of the mid- to caudal abdomen. This mass is causing marked displacement of the small intestinal loops and colon to the right and cranially. There is also dorsal deviation of the descending colon on the lateral view. The abdominal serosal detail within the cranial abdomen is within normal limits with good visualization of the liver margins and a small portion of the spleen, ventral to the mass on the lateral view. The left kidney cannot be identified separate from the mass. Incidentally, spondylosis deformans is present at L203.

2 What is your radiographic diagnosis? Large soft tissue opaque mid-abdominal mass. The most likely differential diagnoses for the origin of the mass would include spleen or left kidney. The most likely differential diagnosis for an intra-abdominal mass, especially one of this size, is neoplasia. Other possibilities could include: abscess, hematoma, or granuloma.

3 Are additional radiographic views needed? An ultrasound of the abdomen could be performed to further characterize the mass. However, when abdominal masses become this large, the origin of the mass can be difficult to determine due to adjacent visceral crowding and compression, even with ultrasound. If further imaging is indicated (i.e. surgical planning), a CT examination may be more beneficial than ultrasound given the size of the mass in this patient. With the concern for neoplasia, a three-view (left lateral, right lateral and ventrodorsal/dorsoventral) radiographic study or CT examination of the thorax would be recommended, looking for evidence of pulmonary metastatic disease.

Final diagnosis: Left renal mass. Histopathologically, this mass was determined to be a metastatic lesion from a left front peripheral nerve sheath tumor, diagnosed approximately 6 months earlier.

CASE 2.16

1 What are your radiographic findings? A soft tissue opaque mass is present in the dorsal caudal abdomen, ventral to the caudal lumbar spine and dorsal to the descending colon, in the region of the sublumbar lymph nodes. The urinary bladder is moderately cranially displaced, suggesting prostatomegaly; however, the margins of the prostate are not clearly defined. The subcutaneous and cutaneous tissues along the caudal ventrolateral abdomen are heterogeneous in opacity and thickened, consistent with known ventral edema and pyoderma.
2 What is your radiographic diagnosis? Marked sublumbar lymphadenomegaly, prostatomegaly.
3 Is additional imaging needed? An abdominal ultrasound could be performed to further evaluate the sublumbar lymph nodes and prostate. Ultrasound could also be used to guide fine needle aspirates for cytology.

Comment: An ultrasound was performed in this case and confirmed the marked sublumbar lymphadenomegaly and an enlarged heterogeneous prostate. Ultrasound-guided fine needle aspirates of the sublumbar lymph nodes, liver, and spleen were obtained and cytologic evaluation revealed abnormal mast cells in all three tissues.
Final diagnosis: Metastatic mast cell neoplasia.

CASE 2.17

1 What are your radiographic findings? Two well-mineralized fetuses are present within the uterus, one to the right of midline and one to the left. The skull of the fetus in the left uterine horn is surrounded by gas opacity. Additionally, irregular, stippled gas opacities are also present within the body of the fetus and the left uterine horn on both projections. The abdominal serosal detail is within normal limits. Also note the development of the mammary glands along the ventral abdomen, which contributes to the soft tissue opacity overlying the abdomen on the ventrodorsal view.
2 What is your radiographic diagnosis? Two full-term fetuses, with one fetus being emphysematous.
3 Is additional imaging needed? Ultrasound is helpful for identification of fetal heart rates if late-term fetal death is suspected and radiographs are not conclusive.

Comment: Radiographic findings suggestive of fetal death include malalignment of bones, collapse or overlap of skeletal structures (most commonly the skull bones), loss of the normal fetal flexion and gas within the uterus, surrounding the fetus, or in the vascular system of the fetus. The gas is caused by devitalization of the tissues and is not immediately evident following death of the fetus.

Final diagnosis: Gravid late-term uterus, fetal death.

CASE 2.18

1 What are your radiographic findings? The right kidney is larger than the left kidney. The left kidney is mildly misshapen. Three small smoothly marginated mineral opaque calculi are present caudal to the kidneys in the retroperitoneal space on the lateral view. Two of these calculi are immediately adjacent to each other, while the third is located further caudally at the level of L5. No calculi are identified within the urinary bladder. The abdominal serosal detail is within normal limits.

2 What is your radiographic diagnosis? Right renomegaly, bilateral ureteral calculi.

3 Is additional imaging needed? Compression of the abdomen using a paddle could be performed to get a better view of the kidneys and ureters (**Fig. 2.18g**). Additionally, ultrasound or contrast radiography (excretory urography) could be used to further evaluate the kidneys, ureters, and urinary bladder. Ultrasound images were obtained. **Fig. 2.18c**, sagittal image: a small hyperechoic, shadowing mineral calculus is present in the mildly dilated left ureter. **Fig. 2.18d**, sagittal image: the left renal pelvis and collecting system are markedly dilated with anechoic urine, leaving only a small rim of renal parenchyma. **Fig. 2.18e**, sagittal image: the right kidney is enlarged and the renal pelvis is dilated with anechoic urine. **Fig. 2.18f**, transverse image: the proximal right ureter is dilated with anechoic urine. Typically, the proximal ureter is small and difficult to identify.

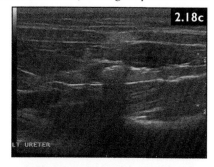

Final diagnosis: Bilateral obstructive nephropathy and hydronephrosis (worse on the left) secondary to ureteral calculi.

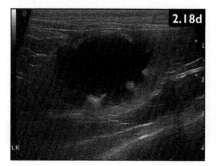

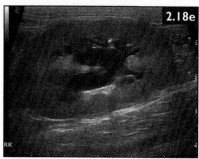

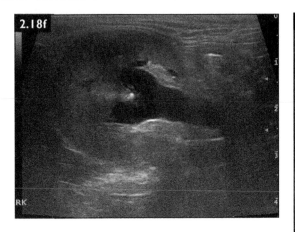

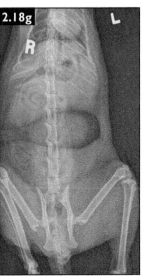

CASE 2.19

1 What are your radiographic findings? Increased soft tissue opacity is present in the right cranial abdomen, causing caudal deviation of the stomach axis and displacement of the intestinal loops to the left and caudally. On the lateral view, the caudal margin of this soft tissue opacity is rounded and extends dorsal to the spleen and ventral to the colon. The liver extends caudal to the costochondral junction, suggestive of enlargement. The abdominal serosal detail is mildly reduced throughout the abdomen.

2 What is your radiographic diagnosis? Right cranial abdominal mass. The most likely differential diagnosis for the origin of the mass is the liver based on the location and caudal deviation of the gastric axis.

3 Is additional imaging needed? An abdominal ultrasound or computed tomography examination of the abdomen could be performed to further evaluate this mass and obtain a diagnostic sample for a more definitive diagnosis. An ultrasound image of the large heterogeneous liver mass is shown (**Fig. 2.19c**).

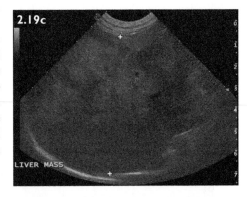

Comment: Differential diagnoses for a hepatic mass include primary and metastatic neoplasia (i.e. hepatocellular carcinoma, biliary carcinoma, adenoma), abscess, granuloma, or an hepatic cyst.

Final diagnosis: Hepatic adenoma.

CASE 2.20

1 **What are your radiographic findings?** The kidneys are ventrally displaced on the lateral view. The margins of the kidneys are difficult to appreciate due to loss of serosal detail within the peritoneal space. The peritoneal detail is also mildly decreased, with small accumulations of gas in the ventral abdomen and subcutaneous tissues, consistent with recent surgery. The duodenum maintains a similar diameter within the right cranial abdomen on both views, suggestive of a focal ileus. The remainder of the small bowel is within normal limits. The spinous processes of the lumbar spine have been removed, consistent with the prior mass removal.

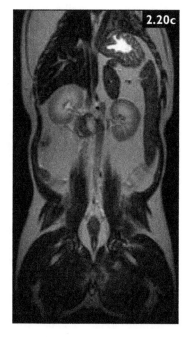

2 **What is your radiographic diagnosis?** Loss of retroperitoneal detail and mass effect. Differential diagnoses include: retroperitoneal fluid (urine or hemorrhage) and/or a retroperitoneal mass (neoplasia, hematoma, abscess).

3 **Is additional imaging needed?** An abdominal ultrasound, computed tomography or magnetic resonance imaging (MRI) of the abdomen could be performed to further evaluate the retroperitoneal space. In this case, an abdominal ultrasound and MRI of the abdomen were performed. An MRI performed 5 days after the initial radiographs (**Fig. 2.20c**, T2 coronal image) shows a heterogeneous contrast-enhancing mass caudal to the right kidney.

Final diagnosis: Metastatic mast cell tumor with surrounding hemorrhage. The diagnosis was obtained from intraoperative impression smears of the mass. Abnormal mast cells were also identified on cytology of the spleen.

CASE 2.21

1 **What are your radiographic findings?** The descending colon contains a moderate amount of fluid, with large bubbles of gas. No formed fecal material is identified. The stomach is empty. The loops of small bowel are normal in size and fluid-filled. The abdominal serosal detail is within normal limits.

2 **What is your radiographic diagnosis?** Fluid-filled colon, consistent with diarrhea.

3 **Is additional imaging needed?** No.

Final diagnosis: Colitis.

CASE 2.22

1 **What are your radiographic findings?** There is a generalized increase in soft tissue opacity diffusely throughout the abdomen, with a loss of abdominal serosal detail. The abdomen is pendulous in shape. Multiple variably sized round foci of gas opacity, which are not definitely associated with the intestinal tract, are distributed throughout the abdomen. No gastrointestinal dilation is evident. Multiple small foci of gas are present along the superficial soft tissues of the ventral abdomen, just caudal to the sternum, consistent with recent abdominocentesis. Incidentally, spondylosis deformans is present throughout the lumbar spine and at the lumbosacral junction.

2 **What is your radiographic diagnosis?** Marked peritoneal effusion and moderate pneumoperitoneum, most consistent with a gastrointestinal perforation or rupture.

3 **Is additional imaging needed?** If free peritoneal gas is suspected in the abdomen, positional radiography, such as a left lateral horizontal beam projection (**Fig. 2.22e**) could be performed. Leaving the patient in left lateral recumbency for 5–10 minutes will allow the gas to rise to the highest point in the abdomen, usually under the

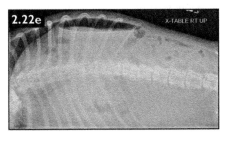

ribs or caudal to the diaphragm. By placing the patient in left lateral recumbency, the gas-filled fundus is ventral and out of the way. Note the moderate amount of free peritoneal gas that accumulates in the nondependent portion of the abdomen, just under the abdominal wall, and does not appear associated with bowel.

Comment: An ultrasound examination was also performed on this patient and a large mass was identified associated with the lesser curvature of the stomach with loss of normal gastric wall layering. At surgery, this was confirmed to be a gastric mass with enlargement of an adjacent lymph node.

Final diagnosis: Metastatic mast cell tumor with secondary peritonitis.

CASE 2.23

1 What are your radiographic findings? A large, smoothly marginated soft tissue opaque mass is present in the mid-abdomen causing displacement of the surrounding viscera. Three large, smoothly marginated mineral opacities are present in the trigonal region of the urinary bladder. The left and right kidneys are normal in margination and in size. A metallic ring (ameroid constrictor) is present in the craniodorsal abdomen, consistent with previous portosystemic shunt ligation. Also of note, the liver is normal in size.

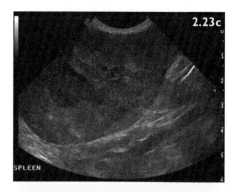

2 What is your radiographic diagnosis? Mid-abdominal soft tissue mass and cystic calculi. Differential diagnoses for the origin of the mid-abdominal abdomen include spleen, lymphatics, and intestines.

3 Is additional imaging needed? An ultrasound or computed tomography

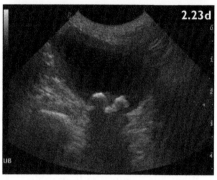

examination of the abdomen would be useful for determining the origin of the mass and for further characterization. Additionally, a fine needle aspirate or biopsy of the mass could be obtained. Ultrasound images obtained in this case are shown (**Figs. 2.23c, d**).

Comment: Ultrasound confirmed the mid-abdominal mass to be spleen (**Fig. 2.23c**). Note the heterogeneity and bulbous appearance of the spleen. Two hyperechoic, shadowing mineral calculi are present in the urinary bladder (**Fig. 2.23d**).

Final diagnosis: Hemangiosarcoma with metastasis to the omentum.

CASE 2.24

1 What are your radiographic findings? The liver is mildly enlarged with rounding of the caudal margins. A marked amount of arborizing mineral opacity is present within the liver. The gastrointestinal tract is within normal limits. No other abnormalities of the abdomen are identified. Incidentally, the lumbosacral intervertebral disk space is collapsed with ventral spondylosis deformans. A mild amount of ventral spondylosis deformans is also present at L1-2.

2 What is your radiographic diagnosis? Biliary mineralization and hepatomegaly.

3 Is additional imaging needed? An abdominal ultrasound could be performed for further evaluation of the liver and biliary system. An image of the mineralization within the biliary tracts is shown (**Fig. 2.24c**).

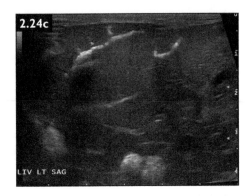

CASE 2.25

1 What are your radiographic findings? Multiple dilated loops of small bowel, filled with gas and fluid, are present within the mid-abdomen. The stomach is moderately gas and fluid distended. The abdominal serosal detail is diffusely decreased. No additional abnormalities are identified.

2 What is your radiographic diagnosis? Small intestinal obstruction.

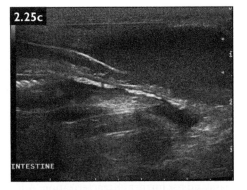

3 Is additional imaging needed? In this case, the small intestinal obstruction can be made with confidence; however, an ultrasound was performed for further evaluation. Note the hyperechoic linear structure within the large, dilated fluid-filled loop of bowel (**Fig. 2.25c**). A loop of small bowel is shown in this image (**Fig. 2.25d**). Note the concentric appearance of this bowel loop.

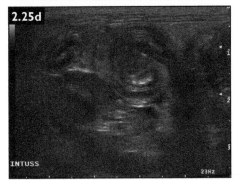

Final diagnosis: Intussusception secondary to a string foreign body.

CASE 2.26

1 What are your radiographic findings? There is a large ventral filling defect within the iodinated contrast pool of the urinary bladder. Iodinated contrast can be seen outside of the bladder, within the peritoneal cavity. Both ureters are clearly seen as are both kidneys.

2 What is your radiographic diagnosis? Large urinary bladder mass; urinary bladder rupture. Mild dilation of the renal pelves and ureters, secondary to obstruction by the urinary bladder mass. The ultrasound image shows the large, solid nature of the mass.

Comment: IVP (or EU) is a radiographic technique that allows excellent visualization of the kidneys (in particular the renal diverticula and pelvis) and ureters. Allowing enough time to elapse to fill the urinary bladder with excreted iodinated contrast results in a positive contrast cystogram. An IVP may then be used to assess the entire upper urinary system and bladder, as opposed to a cystogram alone.

In this case, the renal collecting system is mildly dilated secondary to the large urinary bladder mass. It is usually abnormal to identify the entire length of both ureters, as peristalsis is expected to create 'breaks' in the contrast column.

Final diagnosis: Transitional cell carcinoma with rupture of the urinary bladder and a uroabdomen.

CASE 2.27

1 What are your radiographic findings? The liver is enlarged, extending caudal to the costochondral junction. The spleen is diffusely enlarged. The kidneys are difficult to visualize due to a lack of retroperitoneal fat; however, the left kidney appears small. The stomach is small, containing only a small amount of gas. The loops of small bowel are normal in size, filled with gas and fluid. The colon is normal in size, containing gas and granular fecal material with multiple small mineral opacities. The abdominal serosal detail is diffusely decreased, most severely in the mid-abdomen.

2 What is your radiographic diagnosis? Hepatosplenomegaly, small left kidney, diffuse decrease in abdominal serosal detail.

3 Is additional imaging needed? An abdominal ultrasound would be useful for further evaluation of the liver (**Fig. 2.27c**), spleen (**Fig. 2.27d**), and kidneys and to determine if peritoneal effusion is present.

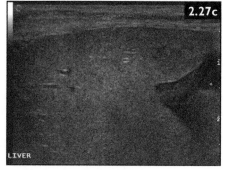

Comment: The most likely differential diagnoses for the enlarged liver and spleen are neoplasia (lymphosarcoma or mast cell disease) or infection. The small left kidney could be associated with chronic kidney disease. The diffuse decrease in abdominal serosal detail may be secondary to the poor body condition of the patient; however, peritoneal effusion should still be considered.

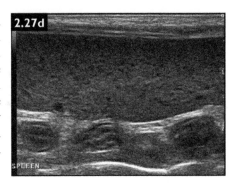

Final diagnosis: Lymphosarcoma.

CASE 2.28

1 What are your radiographic findings? The entire colon is distended and contains a marked amount of mineral opaque, granular fecal material. The remainder of the abdomen is within normal limits with normal serosal detail. On the ventrodorsal view, the caudal lumbar spine curves to the right, consistent with scoliosis. The L5-6 intervertebral disk space is collapsed with partial fusion of the vertebral bodies. The seventh lumbar vertebral body and cranial sacrum are fused. The sacrum is malformed. The caudal vertebral bodies are absent.

2 What is your radiographic diagnosis? Megacolon. Multiple caudal vertebral anomalies (including sacral dysgenesis, absence of caudal vertebrae. and scoliosis).

3 Is additional imaging needed? No.

Comment: Megacolon is defined as a diffuse dilation of the colon secondary to abnormal motility. One of the underlying causes of megacolon is congenital spinal anomalies, common to certain breeds such as the Manx cat. Other differential diagnoses for a megacolon include idiopathic (cats), chronic inflammation or constipation, neuromuscular disorders, trauma, metabolic or endocrine disorders, mechanical obstructions (stricture, lymphadenomegaly, prostatomegaly), or congenital abnormalities.

CASE 2.29

1 What are your radiographic findings? There is a diffuse loss of serosal detail throughout the abdomen. The liver is normal to mildly decreased in size, with mild cranial angulation of the gastric axis on the lateral views. The gastrointestinal structures are normal in size and contain gas and fluid opacity. The urinary bladder is moderately distended. Incidental findings include degenerative joint disease of the hips and spondylosis of the thoracolumbar and lumbosacral spine.

2 What is your radiographic diagnosis? Peritoneal effusion.

3 Is additional imaging needed? An abdominal ultrasound could be performed, primarily evaluating the liver because of the history of elevated liver enzymes, but also to assist in obtaining an abdominal fluid sample. On abdominal ultrasound, a moderate amount of fluid was present diffusely throughout the abdomen. Within the gallbladder, a moderate amount of echogenic debris is present, forming a stellate appearance with small strands

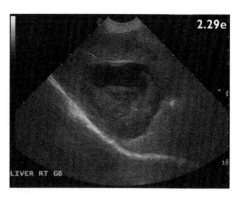

extending to the gallbladder wall (**Fig. 2.29e**). This appearance is most consistent with a gallbladder mucocele.

Final diagnosis: Gallbladder rupture with secondary bile peritonitis. The gallbladder was removed at surgery. On histopathology, the diagnosis of a necrohemorrhagic and ulcerative cholangiocystitis was made.

CASE 2.30

1 **What are your radiographic findings?** Multiple loops of mildly to moderately gas dilated small intestine are present throughout the abdomen, measuring up to 18 mm in diameter. Multiple loops contain a fragmented gas pattern, with gas foci ranging in shape from circular to angular. Within the proximal aspect of the descending colon, there is a focal accumulation of foreign material that has a 'cloth-like' appearance, with linear oriented gas striations and soft tissue opacity. There is a mild generalized loss of serosal margin detail.

2 **What is your radiographic diagnosis?** Small intestinal obstruction, suspect mild peritoneal effusion.

Comment: After stabilization, surgery was recommended for this patient.

Final diagnosis: Small intestinal mechanical obstruction secondary to an intraluminal foreign body.

CASE 2.31

1 **What are your radiographic findings?** A large soft tissue opaque mass is occupying the majority of the mid-abdomen. This mass is causing cranial deviation of the stomach, dorsal deviation of the kidneys, and deviation of the descending colon to the right. No small intestinal dilation is identified. The colon contains a moderate amount of formed fecal material. The liver, kidneys, and urinary bladder can be identified separate from the mass.

2 **What is your radiographic diagnosis?** Large mid-abdominal mass. Differential diagnoses for the origin of the mass include spleen, mesentery, lymph nodes, and/or intestine.

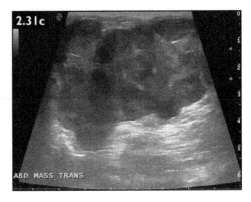

3 **Is additional imaging needed?** An abdominal ultrasound or computed tomography examination of the abdomen could be performed to further evaluate and characterize this mass and determine which structures it may be involving. **Fig. 2.31c** shows a large hetergeneous multilobulated mass throughout the abdomen. An extended field of view image of the mid-abdominal mass (**Fig. 2.31d**) shows a better representation of the full extent of the mass as it spans from the liver to the urinary bladder.

Additionally, fine needle aspirates or a biopsy of the mass could be obtained with ultrasound guidance for a more definitive diagnosis. Thoracic radiographs would also be recommended as neoplasia is a likely differential diagnosis in this case.

Final diagnosis: Lymphosarcoma.

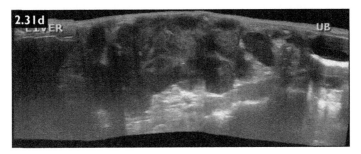

CASE 2.32

1 **What are your radiographic findings?** The gastric axis is deviated cranially, consistent with a reduction in liver size. The gastrointestinal structures are within normal size limits. The descending duodenum is deviated toward midline focally at the level of T12-13 on the ventrodorsal view. Additionally, the serosal detail in the right cranial abdomen is mildly decreased. The urinary bladder is markedly distended; however, no calculi are identified.

2 **What is your radiographic diagnosis?** Microhepatia; loss of serosal detail and mass effect in the right cranial abdomen.

3 **Is additional imaging needed?** An ultrasound of the abdomen could be performed to further investigate the liver and right cranial abdomen.

Final diagnosis: Right cranial abdominal mass, likely originating from the pancreas. An ultrasound-guided fine needle aspirate of the mass was performed and neoplasia (carcinoma) was confirmed on cytology. Differential diagnoses for microhepatia include: variation of normal in deep chested dogs, portosystemic shunting and chronic hepatopathy.

CASE 2.33

1 What are your radiographic findings? A foreign body is identified within a loop of small intestine in the caudoventral abdomen. This foreign body has a tubular shape, with a linear lucent center and undulating, regular lucencies along the periphery, most consistent with a corn cob. On the lateral view, the loop of small bowel adjacent and caudodorsal to the corn cob is abnormally dilated and filled with granular appearing soft tissue opaque material. Several other loops of small bowel cranial to the corn cob are fluid filled and mildly distended. The stomach is normal in size and contains gas and fluid. The colon is difficult to visualize as it is small and contains very little granular fecal material. The abdominal serosal detail is within normal limits.

2 What is your radiographic diagnosis? Small intestinal obstruction secondary to a corn cob foreign body.

3 Is additional imaging needed? Based on location, the corn cob foreign body is most likely to be in a loop of small bowel. However, if the colon is difficult to follow, such as in cases like this, the location of a foreign object within the gastrointestinal tract may be difficult to determine. A pneumocolon can be performed in which the colon is filled with negative contrast (gas) to delineate it from the loops of small bowel. Pneumocolon images from this case, confirming the small intestinal location of the corn cob, are shown (**Figs. 2.33c, d**).

Final diagnosis: Small intestinal mechanical obstruction secondary to a corn cob foreign body.

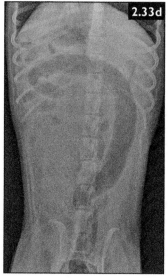

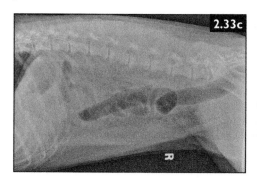

CASE 2.34

1 What are your radiographic findings? Two small mineral opacities are present within the left kidney, which is decreased in size. No abnormalities of the right kidney or urinary bladder are identified. Small metallic hemoclips are present along the midline and to the left of the midline at the level of the left kidney, consistent with the prior adrenalectomy.

2 What is your radiographic diagnosis? Small left kidney with nephroliths.

3 Is additional imaging needed? An abdominal ultrasound could be used to further evaluate the kidneys, ureters, and urinary bladder. A sagittal ultrasound image of the left kidney is shown (**Fig. 2.34c**).

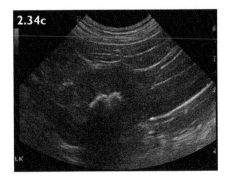

Comment: Visualization of small calculi or mineralization within the kidneys can be difficult due to overlying loops of bowel. A paddle technique or ultrasound examination can be used to help confirm any suspicions.

Final diagnosis: Left nephrolithiasis.

CASE 2.35

1 What are your radiographic findings? The mid-ventral abdominal wall is indistinct. Multiple loops of small bowel are herniated ventrally through the ventral abdominal wall into the subcutaneous tissues. The herniated loops of bowel are normal in size. No subcutaneous emphysema or intraperitoneal gas is identified. The abdominal serosal detail is within normal limits. No fractures or subluxations of the surrounding osseous structures are identified. Incidentally, moderate spondylosis deformans is present at the lumbosacral junction.

2 What is your radiographic diagnosis? Ventral abdominal wall defect and small bowel herniation.

3 Is additional imaging needed? If free peritoneal gas is suspected, a horizontal beam radiograph could be obtained.

Comment: The abdominal wall defect was surgically repaired. At the time of surgery, a lacerated spleen was also identified and removed.

Final diagnosis: Body wall hernia containing loops of small bowel.

CASE 2.36

1 What are your radiographic findings? Multiple markedly distended loops of small bowel are present in the ventral abdomen. The loops of bowel are diffusely filled with a homogeneous soft tissue opacity, likely fluid. Note the few loops of small bowel, with a normal to small diameter, that are present in the caudoventral abdomen, caudal to the distended loops and ventral to the urinary bladder. These loops of small bowel are markedly different in size from the distended loops, which is consistent with two different bowel populations. The stomach is normal in size, containing a small amount of gas and fluid. The colon can be visualized dorsal to the distended small bowel and is normal in size. The colon contains primarily gas and a small amount of fluid, with no formed fecal material identified. Incidentally, both coxofemoral joints have marked degenerative changes, including periarticular osteophytes, irregularly marginated femoral heads and proliferation along the femoral necks. Additionally, smoothly marginated spondylosis deformans is present ventrally at L2-4.

2 What is your radiographic diagnosis? Small intestinal obstruction.

3 Is additional imaging needed? No.

Final diagnosis: Small intestinal mechanical obstruction secondary to a peach pit foreign body. The patient went to surgery to relieve the obstruction.

CASE 2.37

1 What are your radiographic findings? There is a generalized loss of serosal margin detail throughout the abdomen. Additionally, the abdominal contour is mildly pendulous. A moderate amount of heterogeneous soft tissue opaque material is present in the stomach, consistent with a recent meal. The loops of small intestine are primarily gas filled without evidence of dilation. The mid-portion of the descending colon is gas filled with mildly undulating margins. Incidentally, eight lumbar vertebral bodies are present.

2 What is your radiographic diagnosis? Diffuse decrease in abdominal serosal detail. The most likely differential diagnosis is peritoneal effusion.

3 Is additional imaging needed? No.

Final diagnosis: Transudate peritoneal effusion. Intestinal biopsies were performed and a diagnosis of lymphangectasia was made.

CASE 2.38

1 What are your radiographic findings? The liver extends caudal to the costochondral junction and has a rounded caudal margin. The gastric axis is shifted caudally. On the ventrodorsal view, a round soft tissue opacity is present caudal to the stomach, axial

to the spleen, and cranial to the left kidney, which may be a small mass. The loops of small bowel are within normal size limits and filled with gas and fluid. Granular fecal material is present in the colon. The abdominal serosal detail is within normal limits.
2 What is your radiographic diagnosis? Generalized hepatomegaly. Possible small left cranial abdominal mass. Differential diagnoses for the origin of the suspected mass include stomach, spleen, pancreas, or lymph nodes.
3 Is additional imaging needed? An abdominal ultrasound could be performed to further evaluate the liver and possible cranial abdominal mass. Additionally, fine needle aspirates or a biopsy of the liver could be obtained with ultrasound guidance for a more definitive cause of the liver enlargement.

Comment: Differential diagnoses for generalized hepatomegaly could include: vacuolar hepatopathy (i.e. steroid administration, diabetes, Cushings), toxic hepatopathy, cholangiohepatitis andr diffusely infiltrative neoplasia (e.g. lymphoma).
Final diagnosis: An ultrasound of the abdomen was performed. A vacuolar hepatopathy was diagnosed based on a fine needle aspirate and cytology of the liver. A left cranial abdominal mass was also confirmed on ultrasound. A fine needle aspirate of the mass revealed carcinoma, likely originating from the left pancreas.

CASE 2.39
1 What are your radiographic findings? A large filling defect is present on the lesser curvature of the stomach (ventrodorsal view). On the lateral view, the filling defect is seen outlined by a thin rim of barium, void of rugal folds.
2 What is your radiographic diagnosis? Large gastric mass.
3 Are additional radiograph views needed? No.
Final diagnosis: Gastric leiomyoma.

CASE 2.40
1 What are your radiographic findings? Multiple spherical mineral opaque calculi are present in the urinary bladder. Multiple small mineral opaque calculi are also present in the urethra, at the level of the caudal os penis, best visualized on the lateral view with the legs pulled forward. The remainder of the caudal abdomen is within normal limits, with good abdominal serosal detail. Marked spondylosis deformans is present throughout the lumbar spine, including the lumbosacral junction. Marked osteophyte formation is present along both femoral heads and necks. Both acetabula are shallow, with multiple osteophytes cranially and caudally. Irregular mineral opacities are present cranial and caudal to the left and right coxofemoral joints.

2 What is your radiographic diagnosis? Multiple cystic calculi, penile urethral calculi; marked bilateral coxofemoral osteoarthrosis and lumbosacral degeneration.
3 Is additional imaging needed? A contrast urethrogram and cystogram, using iodinated contrast, could be performed to better visualize the calculi, although not necessary for confirmation in this case as the calculi are radiopaque and easily visualized on survey radiographs. A cystourethrogram was, however, performed in this patient to ensure the urethral calculi had been retropulsed into the urinary bladder prior to surgery. A fluoroscopic image following administration of iodinated contrast into the urinary bladder is shown (**Fig. 2.40d**). This highlights the cystic calculi.

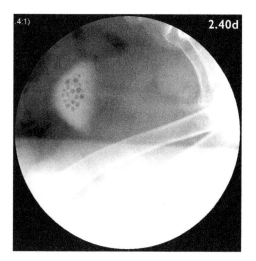

Final diagnosis: Cystic and urethral calculi. Cystotomy was performed to remove the calculi.

CASE 2.41

1 What are your radiographic findings? Multiple variably sized (up to 1 cm) gas opacities are superimposed on the cranioventral hepatic silhouette on the lateral view and just to the right of midline on the ventrodorsal view, in the region of the gallbladder. On both projections, a small mineral opaque structure is present in the region of the right kidney. A linear mineral opacity is present on the lateral view ventral to the L3-4 intervertebral disk space, which may be associated with the urinary system or overlying small bowel. The urinary bladder is moderately distended. A mild decrease in serosal margin detail is present diffusely throughout the abdomen.
2 What is your radiographic diagnosis? Emphysematous cholecystitis, mild peritoneal effusion, right renal calculus.
3 Is additional imaging needed? Based on the location of the gas, an emphysematous cholecystitis is most likely; however, an hepatic abscess compressing the gallbladder could also be considered. Ultrasound confirmed the presence of gas within the gallbladder.

Final diagnosis: Emphysematous cholecystitis. Emphysematous cholecystitis is not very common in canine patients, but can occur secondary to diabetes mellitus, traumatic ischemia, mucocele formation, and/or acute cholecystitis.

CASE 2.42

1 What are your radiographic findings? A large 'mushroom'-shaped crater is present along the antimesenteric border of the proximal-most duodenum. Contrast adheres to this area on the close-up 2-hour radiograph.

2 What is your radiographic diagnosis? Duodenal ulcer; gastric rugal thickening.

Final diagnosis: Zollinger-Ellison syndrome, a rather uncommon syndrome in veterinary medicine. Ulceration is caused by excessive gastrin secretion by a gastrinoma (usually located in the pancreas). Gastrin release by the tumor causes excessive gastric acid secretion by the parietal cells of the stomach. The rugal folds thicken because of the trophic effect of gastrin.

CASE 2.43

1 What are your radiographic findings? There is cranial deviation of the gastric axis and the caudal aspect of the liver does not extend to the costal arch. There is a metal opaque ring within the dorsal cranial abdomen. On the lateral view, there is a soft tissue structure located dorsal to the urinary bladder with very mild narrowing of the descending colon noted. On the ventrodorsal view two oblong soft tissue opaque structures are within the caudal abdomen on either side of midline. The cranial margin of the prostate gland is seen just cranial to the pubis.

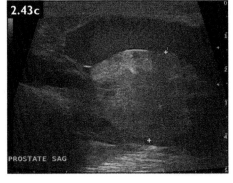

2 What is your radiographic diagnosis? Microhepatia and a caudal abdominal mass, suspected to be originating from the prostate.

3 Is additional imaging needed? Yes. Abdominal ultrasound showed the presence of a complex fluid-filled structure in the caudal abdomen, associated with an enlarged prostate gland and separate from the urinary bladder. An ultrasound image of the prostate surrounded by the hypoechoic fluid-filled cyst is shown (**Fig. 2.43c**). This is diagnostic for a paraprostatic cyst.

Comment: The metallic ring is a vascular occlusion device (amyroid constrictor) used to treat an extrahepatic portosystemic shunt some years ago, which explains the presence of a small liver.

Pathology of surgical specimens confirmed a paraprostatic cyst and prostatic hyperplasia, the latter an expected finding in an elderly intact male dog.

Final diagnosis: Paraprostatic cyst.

CASE 2.44

1 What are your radiographic findings? Two smoothly marginated mineral opacities are present in the left kidney, which is markedly reduced in size. The right kidney is difficult to visualize due to overlying bowel. Two mineralized opacities are also present in the urinary bladder, consistent with cystic calculi. The small bowel is uniformly filled with gas and fluid, without evidence of distension or a small bowel obstruction.

2 What is your radiographic diagnosis? Small left kidney with two nephroliths, cystic calculi.

3 Is additional imaging needed? An abdominal ultrasound or excretory urography could be performed to further evaluate the urinary system. Two ultrasound images from this patient are shown: **Fig. 2.44c**, left kidney; **Fig. 2.44d**, urinary bladder. Note the loss of normal architecture of the left kidney (essentially unrecognizable as kidney between electronic cursors) and the large hyperechoic, shadowing focus of mineral within the renal pelvis. The cystic calculi (between electronic cursors) are also hyperechoic with a dark acoustic shadow, characteristic for mineral.

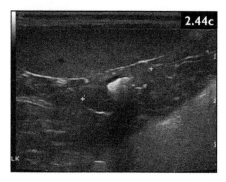
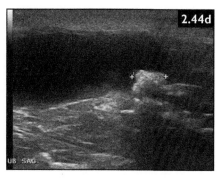

Comment: Normal kidney length in the dog is approximately 2.5–3.5 times the length of the second vertebral body. Chronic kidney disease is the most likely differential diagnosis for a small kidney, especially if the margins or shape of the kidney are irregular. Other considerations for small kidneys include renal hypoplasia, dysplasia, or familial renal disease.

Final diagnosis: Chronic left nephropathy and nephrolithiasis. Cystic calculi.

CASE 2.45

1 What are your radiographic findings? The stomach is air filled, outlining gastric wall mineralization. Mineralization of the kidneys is also present.

2 What is your radiographic diagnosis? Gastric wall mineralization; renal mineralization.

3 Is additional imaging needed? No.

Comment: This case illustrates a dramatic case of gastric wall mineralization. It is a rare complication of chronic kidney disease.

Final diagnosis: Uremic gastropathy. Mineralization or calcification of the gastric wall can occur secondary to chronic kidney disease, as was the case in this patient.

CASE 3.1 A 4-year-old spayed female Chesapeake Bay Retriever with a mass on the left hind foot. You obtain these radiographs of the left hind extremity: **Fig. 3.1a**, dorsoplantar projection; **Fig. 3.1b**, dorsolateral-to-plantaromedial oblique projection.

1 What are your radiographic findings?
2 What is your radiographic diagnosis?

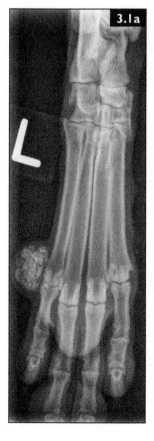
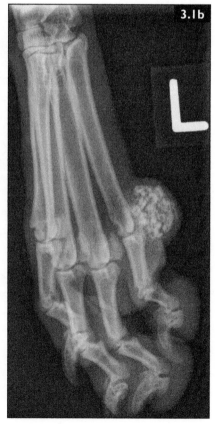

CASE 3.2 A 6-year-old spayed female mixed breed dog with lethargy, anorexia, and diffuse swelling of all four limbs. You obtain these radiographs of the left carpus: **Fig. 3.2a**, lateral projection; **Fig. 3.2b**, dorsopalmar projection.

1 What are your radiographic findings?
2 What is your radiographic diagnosis?
3 What radiographic procedure should be performed next?

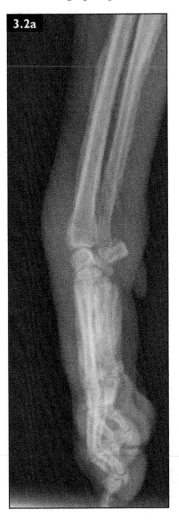
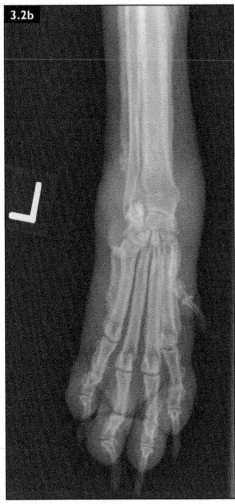

CASE 3.3 A 9-month-old female Labrador Retriever with bilateral forelimb lameness, worse on the right. You obtain this lateral view radiograph of the left shoulder (**Fig. 3.3**).

1 What are your radiographic findings?
2 What is your radiographic diagnosis?
3 Are additional radiographic views needed?

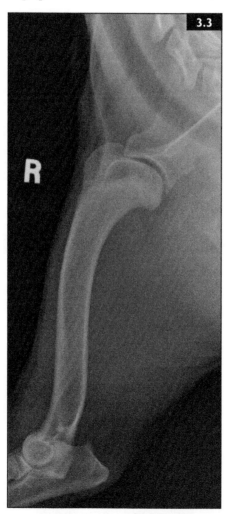

CASE 3.4 A 6-month-old female Labrador Retriever with pain on manipulation of both elbows. You obtain these radiographs of the left elbow: **Fig. 3.4a**, lateral projection; **Fig. 3.4b**, flexed lateral projection; **Fig. 3.4c**, craniocaudal projection.

1 What are your radiographic findings?
2 What is your radiographic diagnosis?
3 Are additional radiographic views needed?

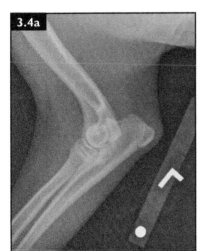

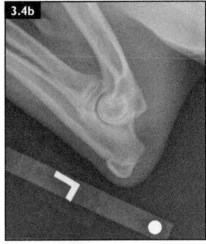

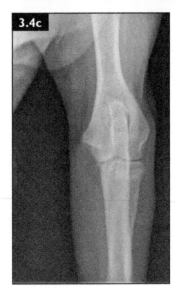

CASE 3.5 A 3-month-old female Labrador Retriever with acute nonweight-bearing lameness in the right hindlimb. You obtain these radiographs of the left stifle: **Fig. 3.5a**, left lateral projection; **Fig. 3.5b**, caudocranial projection.

1 What are your radiographic findings?
2 What is your radiographic diagnosis?

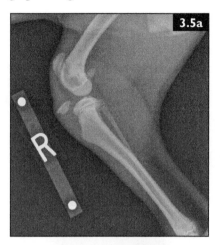

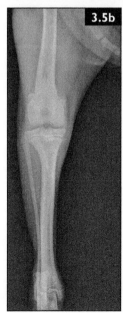

159

CASE 3.6 A 6-year-old male Great Pyrenees with mildly progressive lameness in the right hindlimb; he also seems stiff after exercise. You obtain these radiographs of the pelvis: **Fig. 3.6a,** lateral projection; **Fig. 3.6b,** extended ventrodorsal projection.

1 What are your radiographic findings?
2 What is your radiographic diagnosis?

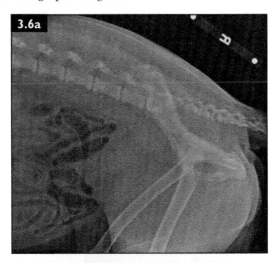

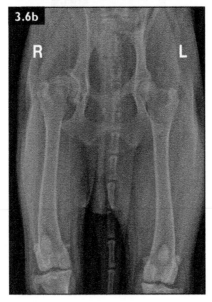

CASE 3.7 A 9-year-old male Labrador Retriever with bilateral forelimb lameness of 6 months' duration. You obtain these radiographs of the shoulders: **Fig. 3.7a**, lateral projection (right); **Fig. 3.7b**, lateral projection (left): **Fig. 3.7c**, skyline projection (both shoulders).

1 What are your radiographic findings?
2 What is your radiographic diagnosis?
3 Is additional imaging needed?

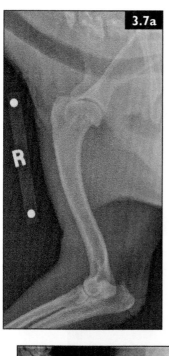
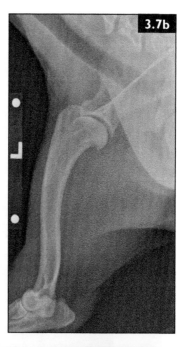
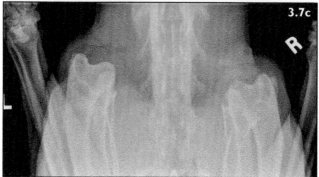

CASE 3.8 A 9-year-old spayed female Labrador Retriever with lameness of the left forelimb for 1 week and a mass palpated dorsal to the left scapula. You obtain these thoracic radiographs: **Fig. 3.8a**, right lateral view of the thorax; **Fig. 3.8b**, ventrodorsal projection.

1 What are your radiographic findings?
2 What is your radiographic diagnosis?
3 Are additional radiographic views needed?

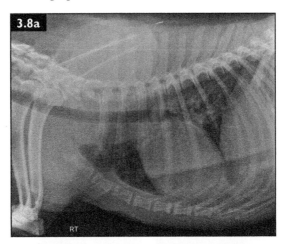

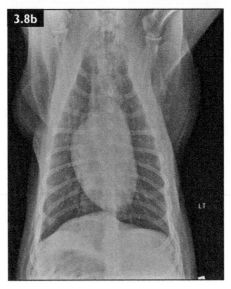

CASE 3.9 A 4-month-old spayed female Labrador Retriever with acute nonweight-bearing lameness in the right forelimb after jumping off a porch. You obtain these radiographs of the right elbow: **Fig. 3.9a,** lateral projection; **Fig. 3.9b,** craniocaudal projection.

1 What are your radiographic findings?
2 What is your radiographic diagnosis?
3 Are additional radiographic views needed?

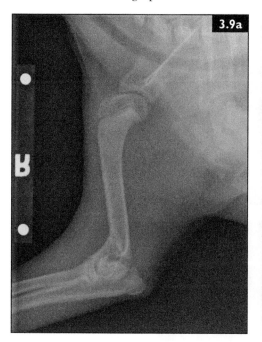
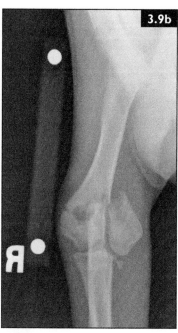

CASE 3.10 An 11-year-old spayed female Labrador Retriever with a history of trauma to the right front second digit and intermittent swelling. You obtain these radiographs of the right front distal extremity: **Fig. 3.10a**, lateral projection; **Fig. 3.10b**, dorsopalmar projection.

1 What are your radiographic findings?
2 What is your radiographic diagnosis?
3 Are additional radiographic views needed?

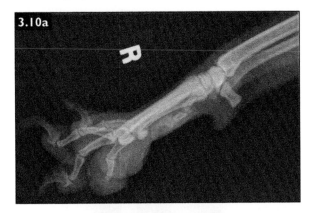

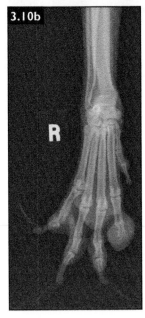

CASE 3.11 A 4-year-old spayed female Belgian Tervuren with right hindlimb lameness and swelling. You obtain these radiographs of the right stifle: **Fig. 3.11a**, lateral projection; **Fig. 3.11b**, caudocranial projection.

1 What are your radiographic findings?
2 What is your radiographic diagnosis?
3 Are additional radiographic views needed?

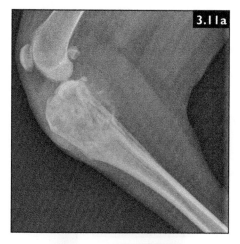

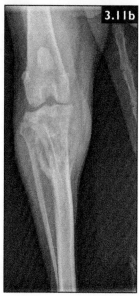

CASE 3.12 A 7-month-old male German Shepherd Dog with acute nonweight-bearing lameness in the right hindlimb. You obtain these radiographs of the right tibia: **Fig. 3.12a**, lateral projection; **Fig. 3.12b**, caudocranial projection.

1 What are your radiographic findings?
2 What is your radiographic diagnosis?

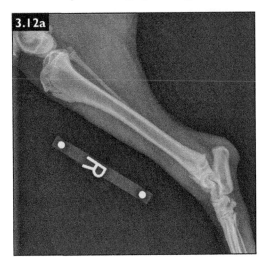

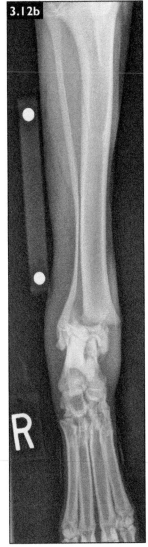

CASE 3.13 A 3-year-old female Shetland Sheepdog with right hindlimb lameness. You obtain these radiographs of the right stifle: **Fig. 3.13a**, lateral projection; **Fig. 3.13b**, craniocaudal projection.

1 What are your radiographic findings?
2 What is your radiographic diagnosis?
3 Are additional radiographic views needed?

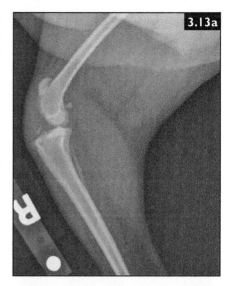

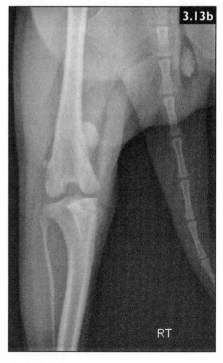

CASE 3.14 A 7-month-old male German Shepherd Dog with acute lameness of the right forelimb. You obtain these radiographs of the right elbow: **Fig. 3.14a,** lateral projection; **Fig. 3.14b,** craniocaudal projection.

1 What are your radiographic findings?
2 What is your radiographic diagnosis?

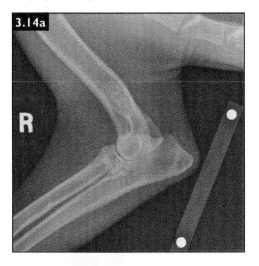

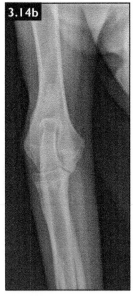

CASE 3.15 A 3-year-old neutered male Labrador Retriever with right forelimb lameness for 6 months. On physical examination, the right carpus has decreased range of motion and is swollen. You obtain these radiographs of the right carpus: **Fig. 3.15a**, lateral projection; **Fig. 3.15b**, dorsopalmar projection.

1 What are your radiographic findings?
2 What is your radiographic diagnosis?
3 Are additional radiographic views needed?

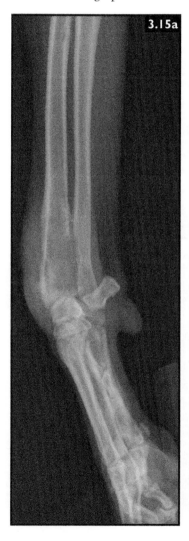
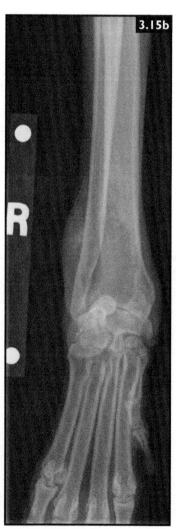

CASE 3.16 A 7-month-old male English Bulldog. Owner reports the dog is reluctant to lift his head or open his jaw. Physical examination reveals facial swelling, right-sided ptosis, myosis, and enophthalmus, with decreased blink and menace reflexes. You obtain these radiographs of the skull: **Fig. 3.16a**, lateral projection; **Fig. 3.16b**, dorsoventral projection; **Fig. 3.16c**, oblique projection.

1 What are your radiographic findings?
2 What is your radiographic diagnosis?

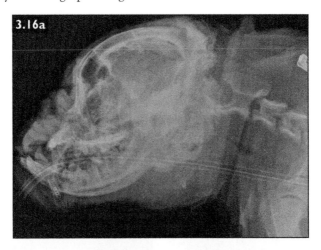

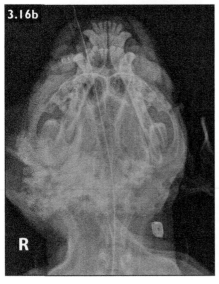

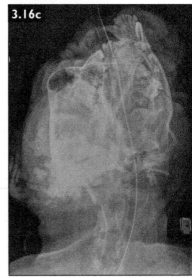

CASE 3.17 A 1-year-old neutered male domestic shorthair cat with chronic right hindlimb lameness. You obtain these radiographs of the pelvis: **Fig. 3.17a**, lateral projection; **Fig. 3.17b**, ventrodorsal projection.

1 What are your radiographic findings?
2 What is your radiographic diagnosis?

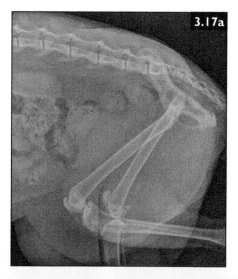

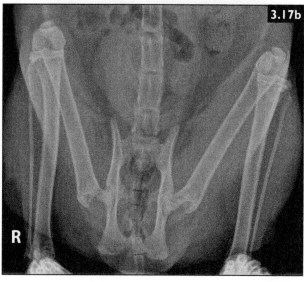

CASE 3.18 A 2-year-old spayed female mixed breed dog with a stiff hindlimb gait. The owner also reports occasional vocalization when playing hard. You obtain these radiographs of the pelvis: **Fig. 3.18a**, lateral projection; **Fig. 3.18b**, extended ventrodorsal projection.

1 What are your radiographic findings?
2 What is your radiographic diagnosis?

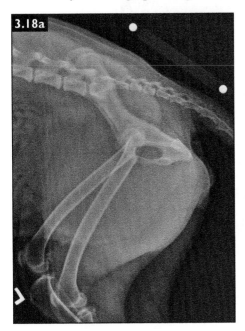

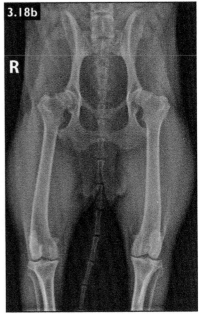

CASE 3.19 A 1-year-old spayed female Basenji with a right forelimb lameness of 2 weeks duration. You obtain these radiographs of the right elbow: **Fig. 3.19a**, lateral projection; **Fig. 3.19b**, craniocaudal projection; **Fig. 3.19c**, flexed lateral projection.

1 What are your radiographic findings?
2 What is your radiographic diagnosis?

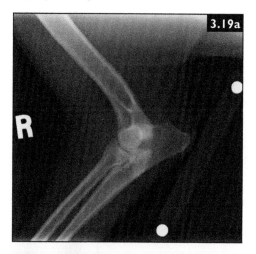

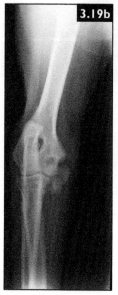

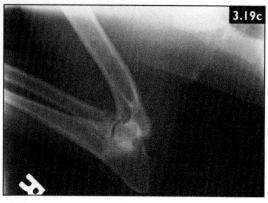

CASE 3.20 A 9-year-old neutered male German Shepherd Dog with acute nonweight-bearing lameness in right forelimb that commenced 2 days ago. You obtain these radiographs of the right humerus: Fig. 3.20a, lateral projection; Fig. 3.20b, craniocaudal projection.

1 What are your radiographic findings?
2 What is your radiographic diagnosis?
3 Are additional radiographic views needed?

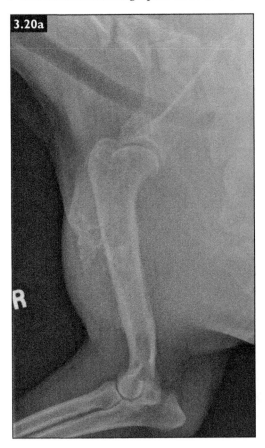

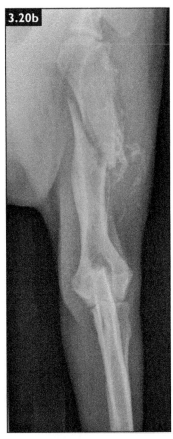

CASE 3.21 A 5-year-old spayed female Golden Retriever who was hit by a car 7 weeks ago. On physical examination, pain is elicited on palpation of the caudal lumbar spine. You obtain these radiographs of the lumbar spine: **Fig. 3.21a**, lateral projection; **Fig. 3.21b**, ventrodorsal projection.

1 What are your radiographic findings?
2 What is your radiographic diagnosis?
3 Are additional radiographic views needed?

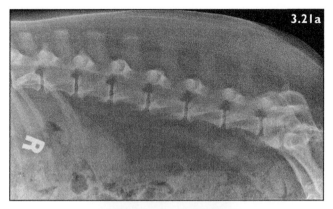

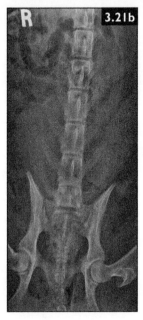

CASE 3.22 A 5-month-old male Great Dane with a left forelimb lameness and swelling of the left elbow. You obtain these radiographs of the left elbow and left carpus: **Fig. 3.22a**, lateral projection left carpus; **Fig. 3.22b**, dorsopalmar projection left carpus; **Fig. 3.22c**, lateral projection left elbow; **Fig. 3.22d**, craniocaudal projection left elbow.

1 What are your radiographic findings?
2 What is your radiographic diagnosis?
3 Are additional radiographic views needed?

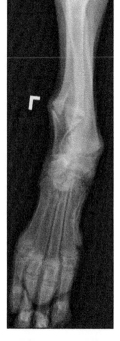

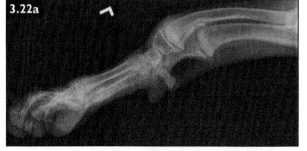

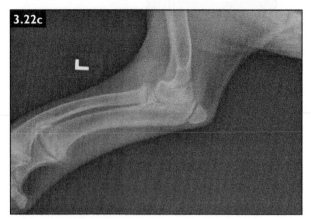

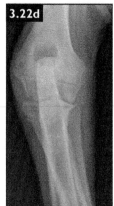

CASE 3.23 A 3-year-old neutered male Labrador Retriever with right hindlimb lameness. You obtain these radiographs of the right tarsus: **Fig. 3.23a**, lateral projection; **Fig. 3.23b**, dorsoplantar projection.

1 What are your radiographic findings?
2 What is your radiographic diagnosis?
3 Are additional radiographs needed?

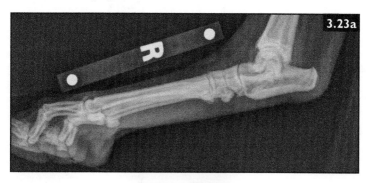

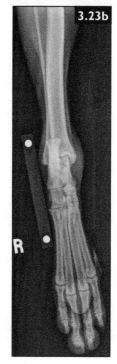

CASE 3.24 A 6-year-old spayed female Labrador Retriever with a left hindlimb lameness. You obtain these radiographs of the left stifle: **Fig. 3.24a**, lateral projection; **Fig. 3.24b**, caudocranial projection.

1 What are your radiographic findings?
2 What is your radiographic diagnosis?

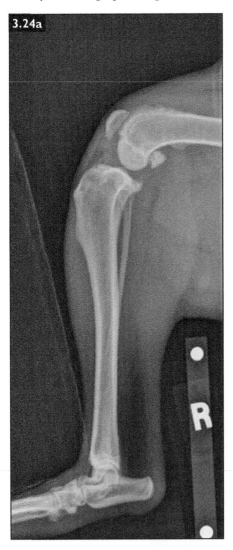

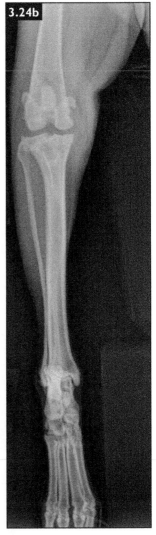

CASE 3.25 A 7 year old neutered male Boxer with a right forelimb lameness and palpable enlargement of the right elbow. You obtain these radiographs of the right elbow: **Fig. 3.25a,** lateral projection; **Fig. 3.25b,** craniocaudal projection.

1 What are your radiographic findings?
2 What is your radiographic diagnosis?
3 Are additional radiographs needed?

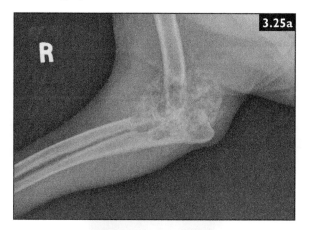

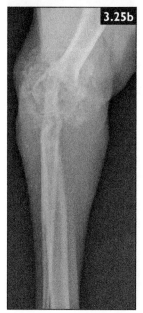

CASE 3.26 A 5-month-old male English Bulldog. The owner reports that the right forelimb looks different from the left forelimb. You obtain these radiographs of the right antebrachium: **Fig. 3.26a**, lateral projection; **Fig. 3.26b**, craniocaudal projection.

1 What are your radiographic findings?
2 What is your radiographic diagnosis?

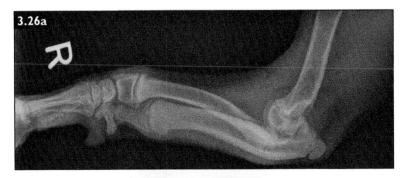

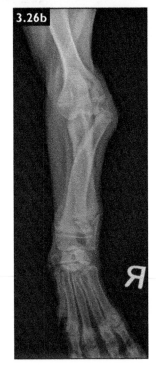

CASE 3.27 A 1-year-old neutered male Rottweiler with bilateral hindlimb lameness and pelvic pain, the left being more severe than the right. You obtain these radiographs of the pelvis: **Fig. 3.27a**, lateral projection; **Fig. 3.27b**, extended ventrodorsal projection; **Fig. 3.27c**, flexed ventrodorsal projection.

1 What are your radiographic findings?
2 What is your radiographic diagnosis?

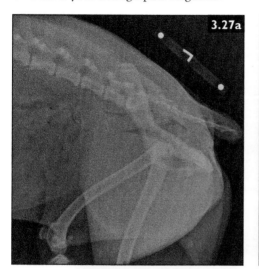
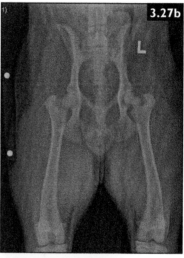
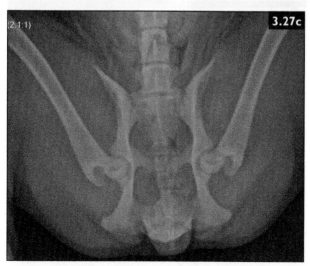

CASE 3.28 An 11-year-old spayed female Labrador Retriever with pain on palpation of the caudal lumbar spine. The owner reports that the dog no longer jumps into the truck. You obtain these radiographs of the pelvis: **Fig. 3.28a**, lateral projection; **Fig. 3.28b**, neutral ventrodorsal projection.

1 What are your radiographic findings?
2 What is your radiographic diagnosis?

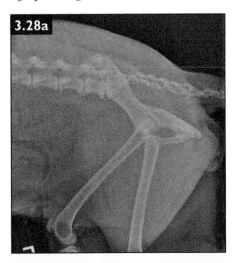

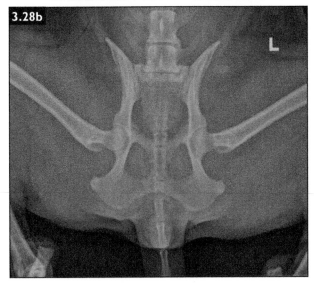

CASE 3.29 A 1-year-old neutered male mixed breed dog with a bilateral forelimb lameness, worse on the right. You obtain these radiographs of the right elbow: Fig. 3.29a, lateral projection; Fig. 3.29b, craniocaudal projection; Fig. 3.29c, flexed lateral projection.

1   What are your radiographic findings?
2   What is your radiographic diagnosis?
3   Are additional radiographs needed?

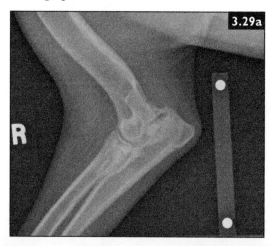

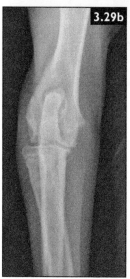

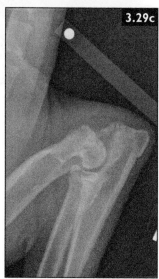

CASE 3.30 A 7-month-old male German Shepherd Dog with lameness in the left hindlimb. You obtain these radiographs of the left stifle: **Fig. 3.30a**, lateral projection; **Fig. 3.30b**, craniocaudal projection.

1 What are your radiographic findings?
2 What is your radiographic diagnosis?
3 Are additional radiographs needed?

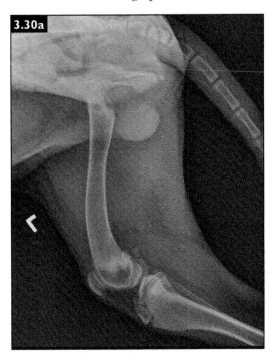

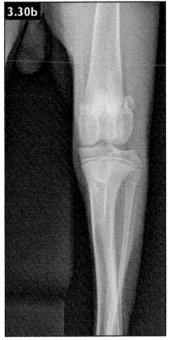

CASE 3.31 A 1-year-old female Great Dane with an enlarged, painful fourth digit. You obtain these radiographs of the left manus: **Fig. 3.31a**, lateral projection (digits spread with the fourth digit positioned dorsally); **Fig. 3.31b**, dorsopalmar projection.

1 What are your radiographic findings?
2 What is your radiographic diagnosis?

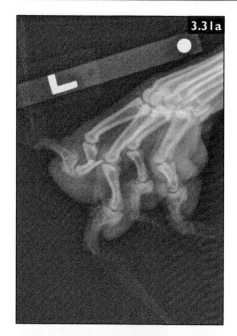

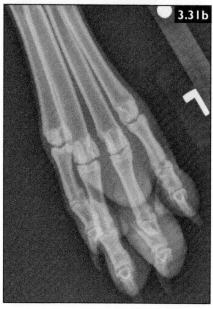

CASE 3.32 A 6-month-old female Labrador Retriever with a lameness that started 2 weeks ago in the left hindlimb. You obtain these radiographs of the left stifle: Fig. 3.32a, lateral projection; Fig. 3.32b, caudocranial projection.

1 What are your radiographic findings?
2 What is your radiographic diagnosis?

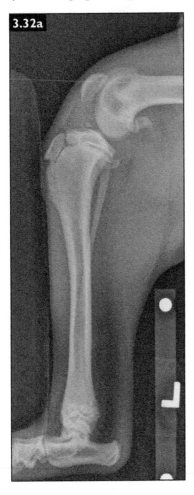
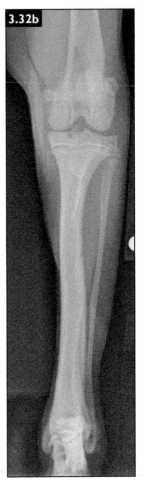

CASE 3.33 A 7-month-old neutered male Rottweiler with bilateral forelimb lameness and pain on palpation and manipulation of the elbows. You obtain these radiographs of the left elbow: **Fig. 3.33a,** lateral projection; **Fig. 3.33b,** craniocaudal projection.

1 What are your radiographic findings?
2 What is your radiographic diagnosis?
3 Are additional radiographs needed?

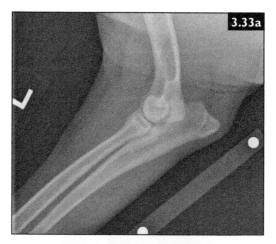

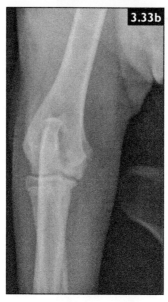

CASE 3.34 A 5-year-old spayed female German Shorthair Pointer with a history of falling out of a truck. You obtain these radiographs of the left stifle: **Fig. 3.34a**, lateral projection; **Fig. 3.34b**, caudocranial projection.

1 What are your radiographic findings?
2 What is your radiographic diagnosis?

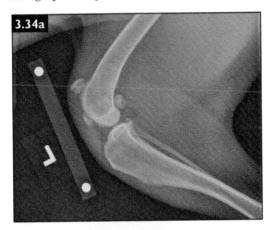

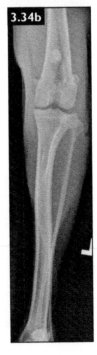

CASE 3.35 A 10-year-old neutered male Viszla with thoracolumbar spinal pain. You obtain these radiographs of the thoracolumbar spine: **Fig. 3.35a**, lateral projection; **Fig. 3.35b**, ventrodorsal projection.

1 What are your radiographic findings?
2 What is your radiographic diagnosis?
3 Are additional radiographs needed?

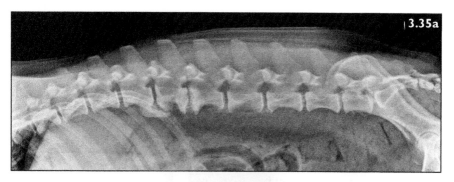

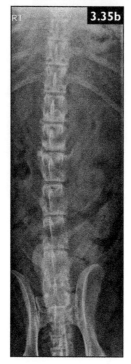

CASE 3.36 A 1-year-old spayed female Boxer with a right hind nonweight-bearing lameness and pain on palpation of the right tibia. You obtain these radiographs of the right tibia: **Fig. 3.36a**, lateral projection; **Fig. 3.36b**, craniocaudal projection.

1 What are your radiographic findings?
2 What is your radiographic diagnosis?

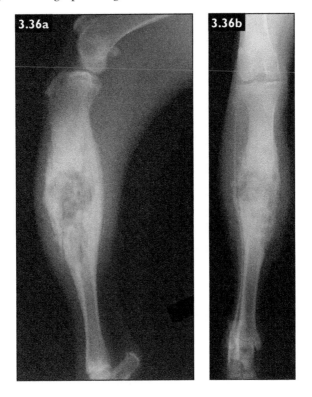

CASE 3.37 A 5-year-old neutered male Labrador Retriever who escaped from the backyard and came home limping on the right forelimb. You obtain these radiographs of the right antebrachium: **Fig. 3.37a**, lateral projection; **Fig. 3.37b**, craniocaudal projection.

1 What are your radiographic findings?
2 What is your radiographic diagnosis?

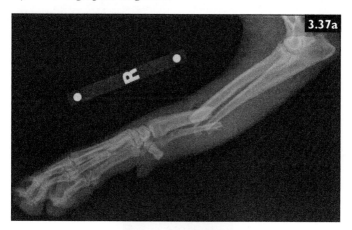

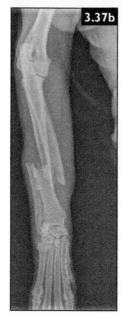

CASE 3.38 An 8-year-old neutered male Basset Hound with paraparesis. You obtain these radiographs of the lumbar spine: **Fig. 3.38a**, lateral projection; **Fig. 3.38b**, ventrodorsal projection.

1 What are your radiographic findings?
2 What is your radiographic diagnosis?

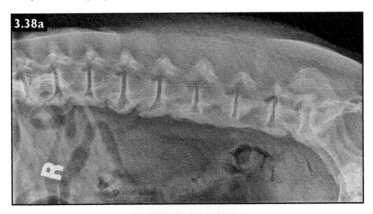

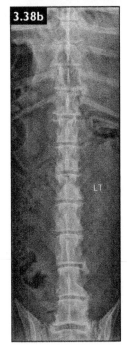

CASE 3.39 A 3-year-old neutered male Australian Cattle Dog with left-sided nasal discharge and epistaxis. You obtain these radiographs of the skull: **Fig. 3.39a,** lateral projection; **Fig. 3.39b,** open-mouth ventrodorsal projection.

1 What are your radiographic findings?
2 What is your radiographic diagnosis?
3 Is additional imaging needed?

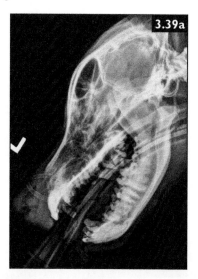

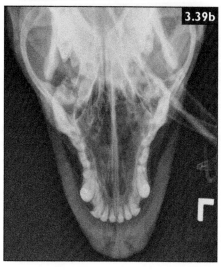

CASE 3.40 A 1-year-old spayed female Pug with right hindlimb lameness and right hip pain. You obtain this ventrodorsal projection radiograph of the pelvis (Fig. 3.40).

1 What are your radiographic findings?
2 What is your radiographic diagnosis?

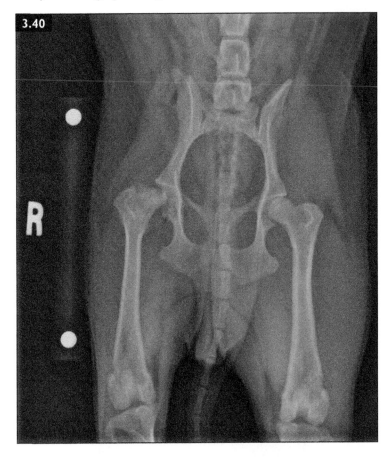

CASE 3.41 A 6-year-old female Collie with an acute right forelimb lameness and carpal swelling. You obtain these radiographs of the right carpus: **Fig. 3.41a**, lateral projection; **Fig. 3.41b**, dorsopalmar projection; **Fig. 3.41c**, stressed lateral projection.

1 What are your radiographic findings?
2 What is your radiographic diagnosis?

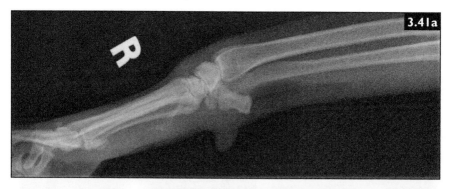

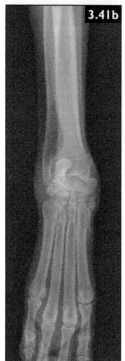

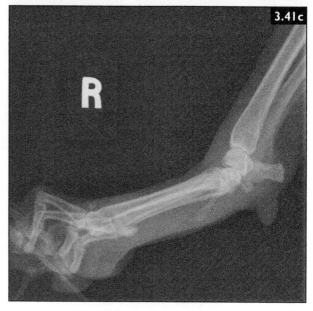

CASE 3.42 A 1-year-old male English Bulldog with a nonweight-bearing lameness of the right forelimb. You obtain these radiographs of the right shoulder: **Fig. 3.42a** lateral projection; **Fig. 3.42b** skyline projection; **Fig. 3.42c** flexed lateral projection.

1 What are your radiographic findings?
2 What is your radiographic diagnosis?

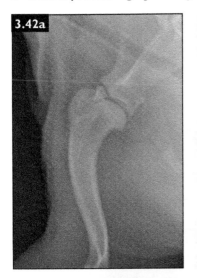

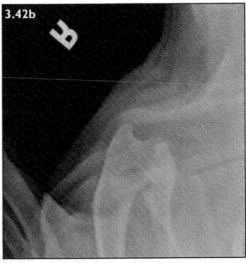

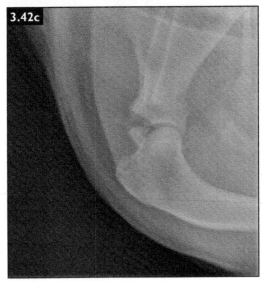

CASE 3.43 A 5-year-old male Miniature Schnauzer with pain and difficulty when walking. You obtain these radiographs of the elbows: **Fig. 3.43a**, lateral projection, left elbow; **Fig. 3.43b**, craniocaudal projection, left elbow; **Fig. 3.43c**, lateral projection, right elbow; **Fig. 3.43d**, craniocaudal projection, right elbow.

1 What are your radiographic findings?
2 What is your radiographic diagnosis?

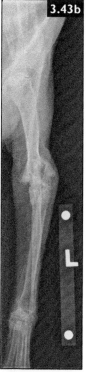

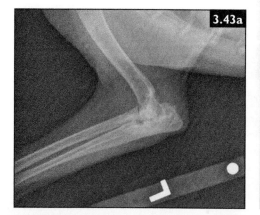

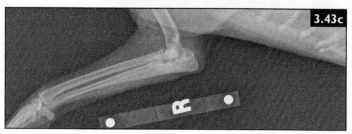

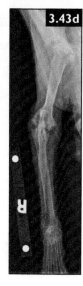

CASE 3.44 A 6-year-old spayed female Catahoula dog with a large palpable mass along the caudal skull. You obtain these radiographs of the skull: **Fig. 3.44a,** lateral projection; **Fig. 3.44b,** dorsoventral projection.

1 What are your radiographic findings?
2 What is your radiographic diagnosis?
3 Is additional imaging needed?

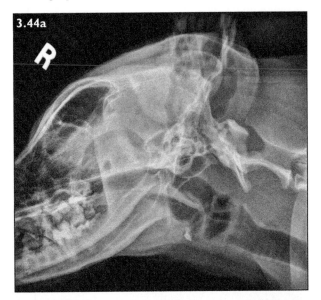

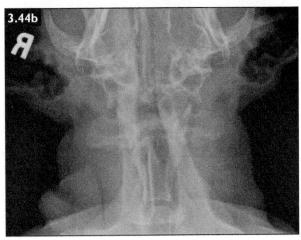

CASE 3.45 A 2-year-old spayed female Labrador Retriever with right tarsal effusion and thickening. No pain on palpation of the limb. You obtain these radiographs of the right tarsus: **Fig. 3.45a,** lateral projection; **Fig. 3.45b,** dorsoplantar projection.

1 What are your radiographic findings?
2 What is your radiographic diagnosis?
3 Is additional imaging needed?

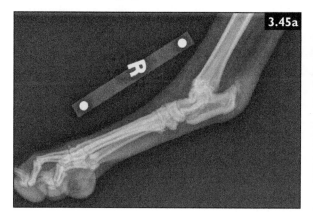

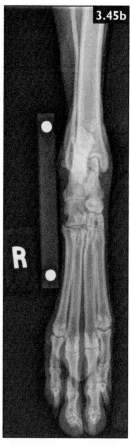

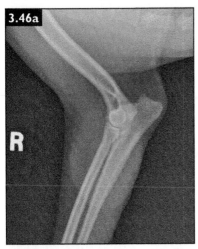

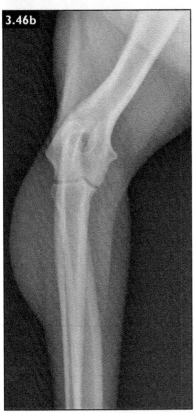

CASE 3.46 A 4-year-old neutered male mixed breed dog with a history of right forelimb swelling. You obtain these radiographs of the right elbow: **Fig. 3.46a,** lateral projection; **Fig. 3.46b,** craniocaudal projection.

1 What are your radiographic findings?
2 What is your radiographic diagnosis?

CASE 3.47 Hindlimb swelling and soreness in a stray dog. You obtain these radiographs of the distal tibia: **Fig. 3.47a**, lateral projection; **Fig. 3.47b**, craniocaudal projection.

1 What are your radiographic findings?
2 What is your radiographic diagnosis?

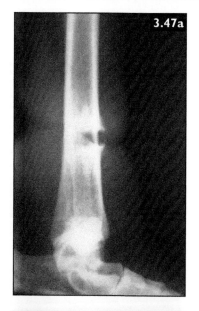

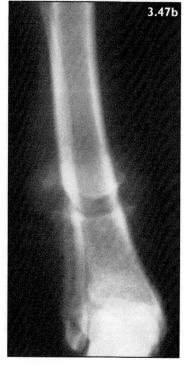

CASE 3.48 A 10-year-old male Schnauzer with paraparesis. You obtain these radiographs of the thoracic and lumbar spine: Fig. 3.48a, lateral projection, thoracic spine; Fig. 3.48b, lateral projection, thoracolumbar spine; Fig. 3.48c, lateral projection, lumbar spine; Fig. 3.48d, ventrodorsal projection, thoracic spine; Fig. 3.48e, ventrodorsal projection, thoracolumbar spine; Fig. 3.48f, ventrodorsal projection, lumbar spine.

1 What are your radiographic findings?
2 What is your radiographic diagnosis?

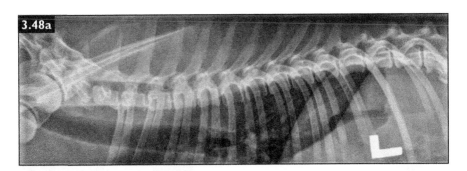

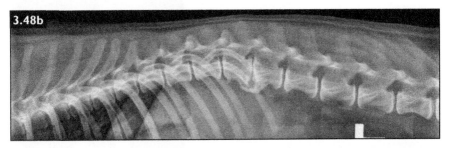

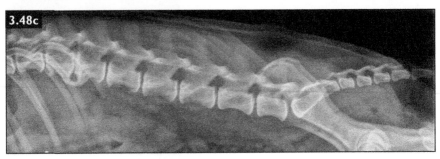

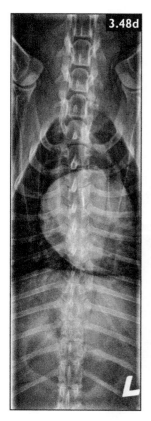

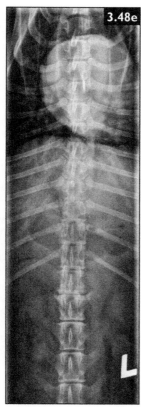

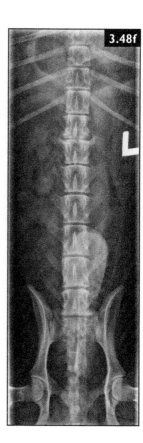

CASE 3.49 A 3-year-old male mixed breed dog who was hit by a car 3 weeks ago. You obtain these radiographs of the pelvis: **Fig. 3.49a**, lateral projection; **Fig. 3.49b**, ventrodorsal projection.

1 What are your radiographic findings?
2 What is your radiographic diagnosis?
3 Is additional imaging needed?

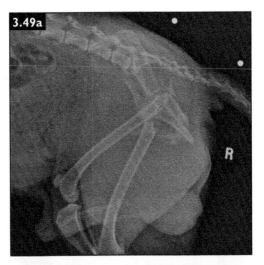

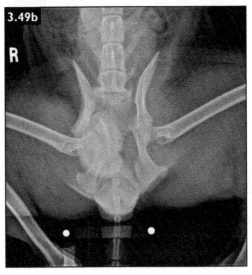

CASE 3.50 A 6-month-old female Bichon Frise with an acute onset of tetraplegia. You obtain these radiographs of the cervical spine and caudal skull: **Figs. 3.50a, c**, lateral projections; **Figs. 3.50b, d**, ventrodorsal projections.

1 What are your radiographic findings?
2 What is your radiographic diagnosis?

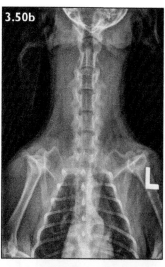

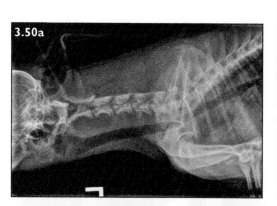

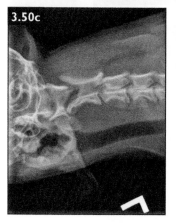

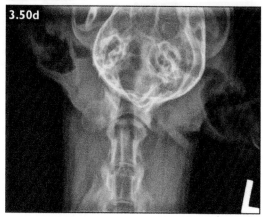

CASE 3.51 A 4-year-old spayed female Border Collie with a chronic fever and a swollen and painful right carpus of 3 weeks' duration. You obtain these radiographs: **Figs. 3.51a, b**, right carpus, lateral and dorsopalmar projections, respectively; **Figs. 3.51c, d**, left carpus, lateral and dorsopalmar projections, respectively.

1 What are your radiographic findings?
2 What is your radiographic diagnosis?

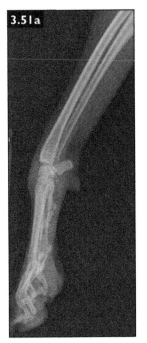
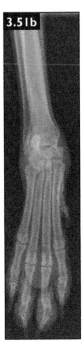
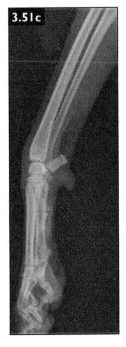
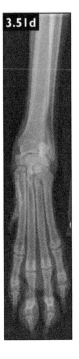

CASE 3.52 A 9-month-old female Borzoi with a history of trauma to the left forelimb. You obtain these radiographs of the left shoulder: **Fig. 3.52a**, right lateral projection; **Fig. 3.52b**, caudocranial projection.

1 What are your radiographic findings?
2 What is your radiographic diagnosis?

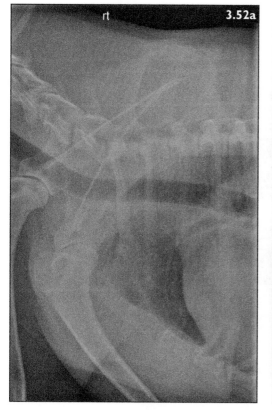
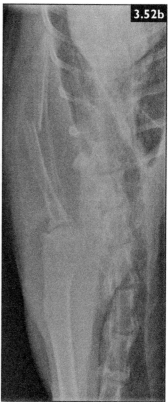

CASE 3.53 A 3-year-old male Weimaraner with a 2-month history of weight loss, loss of muscle mass, and tetraparesis. You obtain these radiographs of the abdomen: **Fig. 3.53a**, Lateral projection; **Fig. 3.53b**, ventrodorsal projection.

1 What are your radiographic findings?
2 What is your radiographic diagnosis?

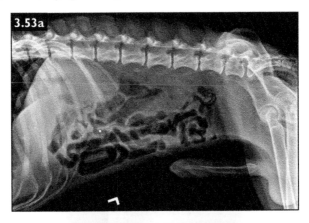

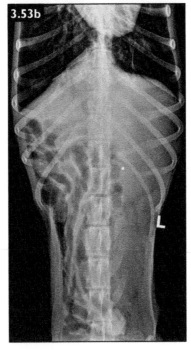

CASE 3.54 A puppy presented for stunted growth and joint stiffness. You obtain these radiographs: **Fig. 3.54a**, shoulder, lateral projection; **Fig. 3.54b**, lumbar spine, lateral projection.

1 What are your radiographic findings?
2 What is your radiographic diagnosis?

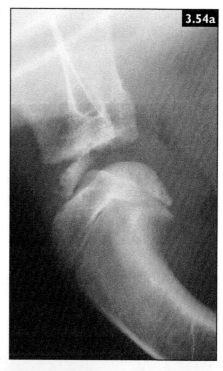

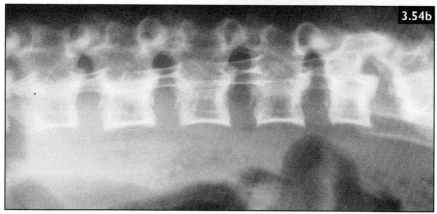

CASE 3.55 A 12-year-old spayed female Golden Retriever who has been licking at the right forelimb. You obtain these radiographs: Figs. 3.55a, b, left carpus, lateral and dorsopalmar projections, respectively; Figs. 3.55c, d, right carpus, lateral and dorsopalmar projections, respectively.

1 What are your radiographic findings?
2 What is your radiographic diagnosis?

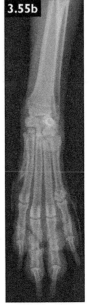

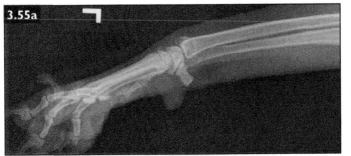

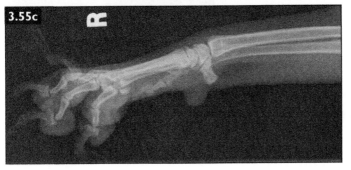

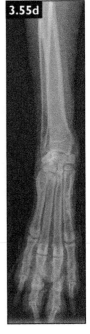

CASE 3.56 A 3-month-old male Australian Sheepdog with a fracture of the left tibia 4 weeks ago. You obtain these radiographs of the left tibia: **Fig. 3.56a**, lateral projection; **Fig. 3.56b**, craniocaudal projection.

1 What are your radiographic findings?
2 What is your radiographic diagnosis?

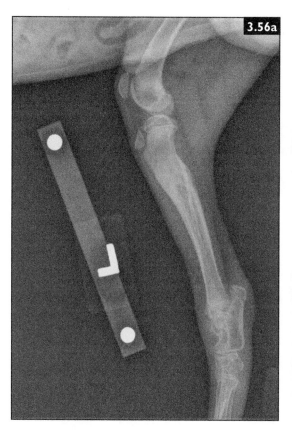
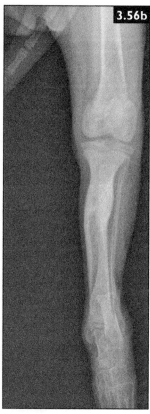

CASE 3.57 An older cat presented for chronic, nonspecific signs of lameness, depression, spinal rigidity, hyperaesthesia, and muscle atrophy. Has been feed a nearly exclusive diet of liver. You obtain these radiographs: **Fig. 3.57a**, cervical spine, lateral projection; **Fig. 3.57b**, thoracic spine, lateral projection; **Fig. 3.57c**, shoulder/elbow, lateral projection.

1 What are your radiographic findings?
2 What is your radiographic diagnosis?

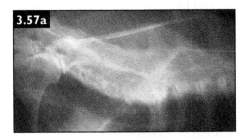

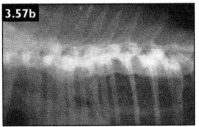

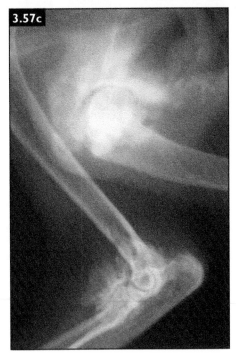

CASE 3.58 An 8-month-old male Yorkshire Terrier with a history of head trauma and difficulty chewing. You obtain these radiographs of the skull: **Fig. 3.58a**, lateral projection; **Fig. 3.58b**, dorsoventral projection; **Fig. 3.58c**, right lateral oblique projection.

1 What are your radiographic findings?
2 What is your radiographic diagnosis?

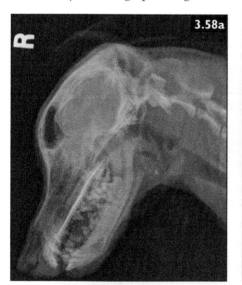

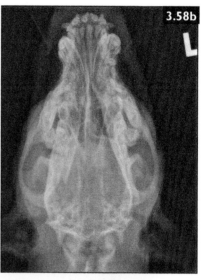

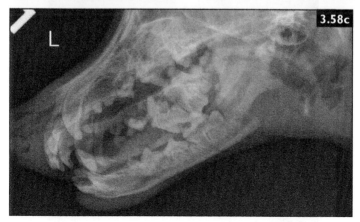

CASE 3.59 An 8-year-old spayed female Labrador Retriever with neck pain that seems to be getting worse. You obtain these radiographs of the cervical spine: Fig. 3.59a, lateral projection; Fig. 3.59b, ventrodorsal projection.

1 What are your radiographic findings?
2 What is your radiographic diagnosis?
3 Are additional radiographs needed?

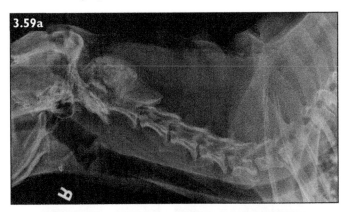

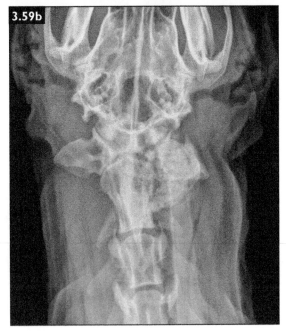

CASE 3.60 A 10-year-old neutered male Dachshund with neck pain for the past 6 weeks. You obtain these radiographs of the cervical spine: **Fig. 3.60a**, lateral projection; **Fig. 3.60b**, ventrodorsal projection.

1 What are your radiographic findings?
2 What is your radiographic diagnosis?

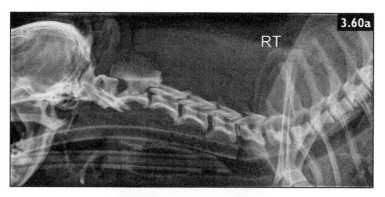

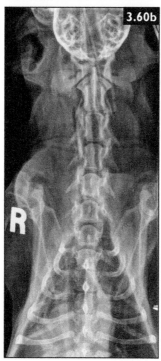

CASE 3.1

1 **What are your radiographic findings?** A smoothly marginated mass, with multiple discrete foci of mineralization, is present along the lateral aspect of the subcutaneous tissues of the left pes, directly adjacent to the 5th metatarsophalangeal joint. The adjacent osseous structures, including the 5th metatarsal bone, first phalanx, and the 5th metatarsophalangeal joint are not affected.

2 **What is your radiographic diagnosis?** Mineralized subcutaneous mass of the 5th digit.

Comment: The lack of adjacent bony reaction on these radiographs indicates a benign, nonaggressive disease process. Calcinosis circumscripta, also known as tumoral calcinosis or calcinosis cutis, is a benign focus of mineralization that occurs within soft tissues. These lesions are found most commonly in the hind foot and oral cavity (i.e. tongue) of the dog and typically seen in young, large breed dogs, such as the German Shepherd Dog. The pathogenesis of calcinosis circumscripta is not entirely understood. Surgical removal is curative.

Final diagnosis: Calcinosis circumscripta.

CASE 3.2

1 **What are your radiographic findings?** Diffuse periosteal reaction is present involving the diaphyseal portions of the radius, ulna, metacarpals I, II, and V, and phalanges of all digits. Note the spiculated appearance of the periosteal response. Soft tissue swelling surrounds the distal limb.

2 **What is your radiographic diagnosis?** Polyostotic periostitis. Differential diagnoses: hypertrophic osteopathy (HO) or infection (hepatozoonosis).

3 **What radiographic procedure should be performed next?** Thoracic radiographs. This patient had diffuse pulmonary metastases from a previously removed osteosarcoma.

Comment: HO is characterized radiographically by mildly irregular to pallisading periosteal proliferation along the diaphysis of long bones in the extremities, with occasional joint involvement. It typically involves multiple bones and can occur in the forelimbs and hindlimbs concurrently. It begins distally and advances proximally as the disease progresses. HO is associated with chronic inflammatory or neoplastic lesions, usually in the thoracic cavity, which is why it is sometimes referred to as hypertrophic pulmonary osteopathy. If the underlying disease can be treated (e.g. excision of a primary lung tumor), the periostitis will often recede.

Periosteal new bone formation, similar to HO, is also a feature of an uncommon protozoon disease in dogs, *Hepatozoon*. This protozoan is spread via tick vectors and found in the south-central and south-eastern United States. The lesions are

217

primarily in the diaphyses of the more proximal long bones, and possibly involve the axial skeleton (vs. HO, which starts distally). Curiously, *H. americanum* is the more common species of *Hepatozoon* to be associated with periosteal reactions, in comparison to *H. canis*. Diagnosis of infection can be through blood smears, muscle biopsies, serology, or polymerase chain reaction tests.

Final diagnosis: Hypertrophic osteopathy.

CASE 3.3

1 What are your radiographic findings? The contour of the caudal humeral head is flattened. A shallow concave defect is present in the subchondral bone of the caudal humeral head. Increased bone opacity, consistent with sclerosis, is present in the subchondral bone deep to the concave defect. The caudal aspect of the glenoid cavity is mildly rounded, associated with early osteophyte formation.

2 What is your radiographic diagnosis? Osteochondrosis of the caudal humeral head.

3 Are additional radiographic views needed? A lateral view of the contralateral limb should be obtained, as osteochondrosis is typically a bilateral condition. Additionally, supinated and pronated lateral projections of the shoulder could be obtained for further assessment in cases where the lesion is not apparent on the straight medial to lateral projection.

Comment: Osteochondrosis is typically found in young, large breed dogs. The caudal humeral head is the most common location for osteochondrosis in the shoulder and best visualized on the mediolateral radiographic projection. The radiographic findings associated with osteochondrosis in the shoulder are a flattened contour or concavity in the subchondral bone of the caudal humeral head, often with underlying sclerosis. Occasionally, a mineralized flap of cartilage along the caudal humeral head can be identified on radiographs. However, if the cartilage flap is not mineralized, it silhouettes with the joint fluid and is difficult to appreciate. An arthrogram (injection of iodinated contrast into the joint) could be performed to help determine if a nonmineralized flap is present, as contrast would be visualized to dissect between the flap and subchondral bone.

Final diagnosis: Osteochondrosis, caudal humeral head.

CASE 3.4

1 What are your radiographic findings? The medial aspect of the coronoid process of the proximal ulna is mildly blunted on the craniocaudal view and indistinct on the lateral view. A mild amount of subchondral sclerosis is present along the trochlea of the distal humeral condyle. Very small osteophytes are present along the cranioproximal aspect of the radial head.

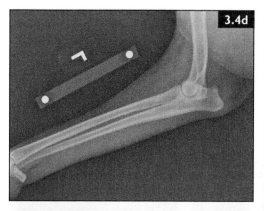

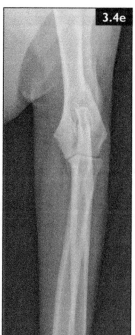

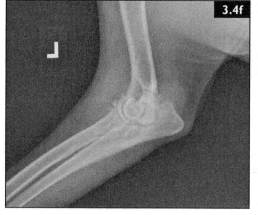

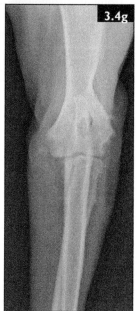

2 What is your radiographic diagnosis? Left elbow dysplasia with medial coronoid disease and minimal secondary osteoarthrosis. An example of a normal medial coronoid process is shown (**Figs. 3.4d, e**). The medial coronoid process should be sharply marginated and distinctly visualized on both radiographic projections.

3 Are additional radiographic views needed? No.

Comment: An example of severe degenerative joint disease in the left elbow, also secondary to elbow dysplasia (medial coronoid disease), is also shown (**Figs. 3.4f, g**). Note the marked osteophyte formation on the medial and lateral distal humeral epicondyles,

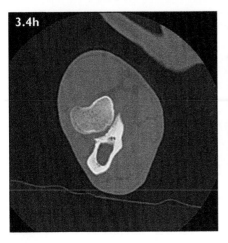

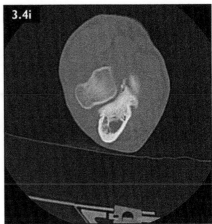

cranial distal humerus, proximal aspect of the anconeal process of the ulna, and cranioproximal radius. The medial aspect of the coronoid process is markedly blunted on the craniocaudal view and indistinct on the lateral view. The articular surfaces of the elbow are undulating in contour. There is also sclerosis of the trochlear notch of the ulna. An irregularly marginated osseous body is adjacent to the medial humeral epicondyle. The soft tissues surrounding the elbow are swollen.

Computed tomography (CT) images are useful for further assessment of the elbow joints, especially in cases of elbow dysplasia. The findings on the CT images are usually worse than the degree of change visualized radiographically. CT also allows for visualization of small fragments adjacent to the medial coronoid process (**Figs. 3.4h, i**), which may not be detected on radiographs.

Final diagnosis: Elbow dysplasia, medial coronoid disease, and osteoarthrosis.

CASE 3.5

1 What are your radiographic findings? The right tibial tuberosity is markedly displaced from the proximal tibia, in a cranial and proximal direction. Several small mineral fragments are adjacent to the cranioproximal tibia and tibial tuberosity. The patella is located more proximal than normal along the femoral trochlea. Soft tissue swelling is present along the cranial aspect of the proximal tibia and in the region of the patellar ligament.

2 What is your radiographic diagnosis? Right tibial tuberosity avulsion fracture.

Comment: In the dog, fusion of the tibial tuberosity with the proximal tibial epiphysis occurs between 6 and 10 months of age and the physis closes between approximately 10 and 13 months of age (can be up to 18 months in large/giant breed dogs). Avulsion fractures can range from widening of the physis to severe displacement of the tuberosity, as seen in this case. Treatment is often conservative for minimally displaced fractures and surgical reduction for more severely displaced fractures.

Final diagnosis: Avulsion fracture of the tibial tuberosity.

CASE 3.6

1 What are your radiographic findings? A marked amount of osteophyte formation is present along the cranial, caudal, and dorsal margins of the right acetabulum. Sclerosis is present within the subchondral bone of the right acetabulum. The right acetabulum is shallow with subluxation of the femoral head. The right femoral head is misshapen with an undulating articular margin and large blunted osteophyte caudally. The right femoral neck is thickened with a moderate amount of osteophyte formation. Also note the decrease in soft tissue opacity along the right hindlimb when compared with the left, which is consistent with muscle atrophy.

2 What is your radiographic diagnosis? Right hip dysplasia, with moderate to severe secondary coxofemoral osteoarthrosis and right hindlimb muscle atrophy.

Comment: Canine hip dysplasia (CHD) is most commonly seen in large breed dogs such as German Shepherd Dogs, Golden Retrievers, Rottweilers, and Saint Bernards. CHD is often a bilateral condition; however, one joint may be more severely affected than the other. The most common radiographic findings of CHD are joint incongruity with possible subluxation and secondary signs of osteoarthrosis (i.e. osteophyte formation, sclerosis, thickening of the femoral neck) later in the course of the disease. Dogs used for breeding are commonly screened for joint laxity, indicative of CHD, at an early age. The two most commonly used radiographic screening methods are the OFA (Orthopedic Foundation for Animals) extended ventrodorsal view or the PennHip distraction method. The radiographic positioning for evaluation of CHD, especially in young dogs, is crucial as slight obliquity could hinder detection of mild incongruity.

Final diagnosis: Hip dysplasia, unilateral.

CASE 3.7

1 What are your radiographic findings? Marked enthesophyte formation is present along the greater tubercle of the proximal humerus, in the region of the supraspinatus insertion, bilaterally. Osseous proliferation is also present bilaterally along the intertubercular groove, best visualized on the skyline view and worse on the right. On the right, the intertubercular proliferation extends both axially and abaxially; however, it is only present along the medial aspect of the greater tubercle on the left. Osteophytes are present along the left and right caudal glenoid cavities and humeral heads, consistent with osteoarthritis.

2 What is your radiographic diagnosis? Bilateral enthesophyte formation at the insertion of the supraspinatus tendon; bilateral intertubercular osseous proliferation, likely associated with bicipital tenosynovitis; bilateral shoulder osteoarthritis.

3 Is additional imaging needed? Often, mineralization within the supraspinatus tendon or enthesophyte formation at the tendinous insertion are the only radiographically evident abnormalities in dogs with supraspinatus tendonopathy. Additional imaging, such as ultrasound or magnetic resonance imaging, of the tendon could be performed to further evaluate the degree of damage to the tendon fibers and size of the tendon.

These axial proton density magnetic resonance images of the left (**Fig. 3.7d**) and right (**Fig. 3.7e**) shoulder from this patient demonstrate bilateral supraspinatus tendinopathy. Note the lack of identification of the biceps tendon on the right, consistent with complete disruption of the tendon fibers.

Final diagnosis: Bilateral supraspinatus tendinopathy with rupture of the right biceps tendon.

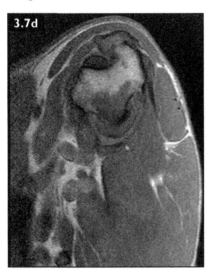 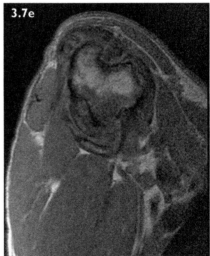

CASE 3.8

1 What are your radiographic findings? On the ventrodorsal view, there is an osteolytic, expansile lesion involving the left lateral scapula. Soft tissue swelling is also present lateral to the left scapula. Incidentally, a fat opaque mass is present lateral to the right scapula, most consistent with a subcutaneous lipoma. The cardiopulmonary structures are within normal limits, with no evidence of pulmonary metastatic disease.

2 What is your radiographic diagnosis? Expansile, osteolytic lesion of the left scapula, most consistent with neoplasia.

3 Are additional radiographic views needed? Right lateral oblique views of the left scapula will allow for better evaluation of the scapular lesion (**Figs. 3.8c, d**).

Final diagnosis: Osteosarcoma, left scapula.

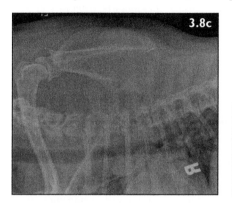

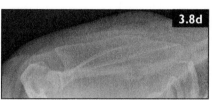

CASE 3.9

1 What are your radiographic findings? There is a Y-shaped condylar fracture of the distal humerus extending through the medial and lateral distal metaphyseal cortices. The large medial fragment is proximally and medially displaced. A small minimally displaced fracture fragment is present adjacent to the medial aspect of the coronoid process of the proximal ulna. Soft tissue swelling is present surrounding the distal humerus.

2 What is your radiographic diagnosis? Type IV Salter–Harris fracture of the distal right humeral condyle; fracture of the medial coronoid process of the proximal ulna.

3 Are additional radiographic views needed? On craniocaudal radiographs of puppies, a small fissure can be visualized between the medial and lateral epicondyles of the distal humerus, which should fuse between 8 and 12 weeks of age. In some breeds, most notably Spaniels, this fissure persists and is termed incomplete ossification of the humeral condyle, which has a potential to predispose these dogs to humeral condylar fractures.

Comment: Fractures of the distal humeral condyle can be classified as medial condylar, lateral condylar, or intercondylar. Intercondylar fractures are further divided into 'Y'-shaped fractures with oblique fracture lines through the medial and lateral metaphysis or 'T'-shaped fractures with more transversely oriented fractures through the metaphyses.

Final diagnosis: Right humeral condylar fracture.

CASE 3.10

1 What are your radiographic findings? Marked soft tissue swelling is present surrounding the distal aspect of the second digit. The third phalanx is no longer present, except for a small faintly mineralized portion of the ungual crest. The distal dorsomedial aspect of the second phalanx of the second digit is irregular with loss of bone opacity, consistent with osteolysis. Incidentally, osteophytes are present along the distal interphalangeal joint of the first digit.

2 What is your radiographic diagnosis? Severe osteolysis of the third phalanx and distomedial second phalanx of the second digit with marked soft tissue swelling. Based on the severity of the osteolysis, the primary differential diagnosis is subungual neoplasia.

3 Are additional radiographic views needed? A three-view (left lateral, right lateral, and ventrodorsal/dorsoventral) radiographic study of the thorax should be performed, looking for evidence of pulmonary metastatic disease.

Comment: The most common tumor of the distal phalanx in dogs is squamous cell carcinoma, followed by melanoma, mast cell tumor, and osteosarcoma. Osteolytic lesions of the distal phalanx can be due to neoplasia or osteomyelitis and these two conditions are often difficult to differentiate radiographically. Biopsy or amputation of the toe is typically performed to determine a definitive diagnosis histopathologically.
Final diagnosis: Squamous cell carcinoma.

CASE 3.11

1 What are your radiographic findings? There is a primarily lytic, expansile lesion of the proximal right tibial metaphysis extending proximally to the subchondral bone. This lesion is causing loss of normal bone trabeculation and thinning of the adjacent cortical bone. A moderate amount of spiculated periosteal proliferation is present circumferentially along the proximal tibia. Also of note, on the caudocranial view, the periosteum along the distal aspect of the lesion appears to be lifted away from the bone. This is known as Codman's triangle and is often seen with aggressive bone lesions. A moderate amount of soft tissue swelling is present surrounding the proximal tibia. The distal femur appears unaffected.

2 What is your radiographic diagnosis? Aggressive, primarily osteolytic lesion of the proximal right tibial metaphysis, most consistent with osseous neoplasia.

3 Are additional radiographic views needed? A three-view (left lateral, right lateral, and ventrodorsal/dorsoventral) radiographic study of the thorax should be performed, looking for evidence of pulmonary metastatic disease.

Comment: Primary osseous neoplasia can be characterized radiographically by osteolysis, osseous proliferation, or a combination of lysis and bony production. Osteosarcoma is most commonly found in the metaphyseal region of long bones;

however, it can involve the epiphysis or diaphysis of the bone. Lesions in the proximal tibia are more common than those in the distal tibia, although both do occur. An example of osteosarcoma in the distal tibia is shown (**Figs. 3.11c, d**).

Final diagnosis: Osteosarcoma.

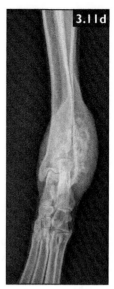

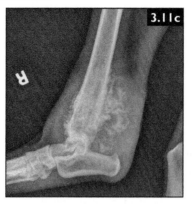

CASE 3.12

1 What are your radiographic findings? There is a cranially and laterally displaced fracture through the right distal tibial physis. This fracture extends through the lateral metaphyseal cortex, leaving a small fragment of metaphyseal bone still attached to the epiphyseal bone laterally. Small bony fragments are present adjacent the fracture. Soft tissue swelling is present surrounding the distal tibia.

2 What is your radiographic diagnosis? Type II Salter–Harris fracture of the distal right tibia.

Comment: Fractures involving the physis in young animals are termed Salter–Harris fractures and adhere to a classification system ranging from I to V. The classification system is based on involvement of physis alone or extension of the fracture into the metaphysis or epiphysis. A type II Salter–Harris fracture is a nonarticular fracture involving the physis and extending into the metaphysis. Types I and V involve only the physis, with type V characterized as a crush injury to the physis. Types III and IV are articular fractures, both extending from the physis through the epiphysis; however, type IV also extends through the metaphysis.

Final diagnosis: Distal tibial physeal fracture (Salter–Harris type II).

CASE 3.13

1 What are your radiographic findings? The patella is medially luxated. The trochlear ridges are mildly flattened in contour. Multiple round and irregularly-shaped mineral opacities are present cranial and proximal to the tibial tuberosity. The tibial tuberosity is misshapen. Increased soft tissue opacity is present along the cranial stifle, with loss of distinction between the patellar ligament and infrapatellar fat pad.

2 What is your radiographic diagnosis? Right medially luxated patella with fragmentation of the tibial tuberosity.

Comment: Luxation of the patella is most commonly diagnosed in small, toy breed dogs; however, it can also occur in large breeds. Luxating patellas can be a congenital problem or occur as a result of trauma. Repeated patellar luxation, or a luxation left untreated, often results in secondary osteoarthritis of the stifle joint.

Final diagnosis: Medial patellar luxation.

CASE 3.14

1 What are your radiographic findings? A patchy focal area of increased bone opacity is present within the medullary cavity of the distal humeral diaphysis. Small foci of intramedullary bone opacites are also present in the proximal ulna. No abnormalities of the elbow joint are identified.

2 What is your radiographic diagnosis? Medullary sclerosis of the distal humerus and proximal ulna, most consistent with panosteitis.

Comment: Panosteitis is a self-limiting condition with an unknown etiology that classically affects the diaphysis of long bones, commonly near the nutrient foramen. It is primarily seen in young (5–18 months), large breed dogs (i.e. German Shepherd Dogs). Radiographically, a patchy increase in opacity of the medullary cavity of

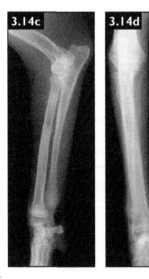

long bones is the most common appearance. In some dogs, smooth endosteal, and possibly periosteal, proliferation is also present along the diaphysis. Radiographic lesions may be present in multiple bones simultaneously, and clinical signs may not always correlate with the presence of radiographic abnormalities.

Another radiographic example of the disease is shown (**Figs. 3.14c, d**, right antebrachium). This patient, another young German Shepherd Dog, exhibited the common presenting complaint of shifting leg lameness, Radiographically, intramedullary opacity is visualized within the proximal and mid-diaphysis of the radius and, to a much lesser extent, the proximal ulna and distal humerus.

Final diagnosis: Panosteitis

CASE 3.15

1 What are your radiographic findings? A large smoothly marginated, osteolytic lesion is present in the distal right radial metaphysis. This lesion extends distally to the subchondral bone; however, it does not appear to affect the radiocarpal joint. The lesion also extends proximally into the distal radial diaphysis, characterized by smaller areas of punctate lysis. There is indistinction of the caudal and lateral distal radial cortical bone and thinning of the cranial distal radial cortex. A mild amount of amorphous periosteal proliferation is present along the lateral and cranial distal radius. A mild amount of smoothly-marginated periosteal proliferation is extending along the cranioproximal distal radial metaphysis and diaphysis. Soft tissue swelling is present surrounding the distal radius. The carpus does not appear affected.

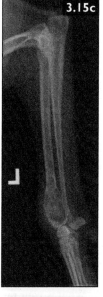

2 What is your radiographic diagnosis? Osteolytic lesion of the distal right radius, most consistent with primary osseous neoplasia.

3 Are additional radiographic views needed? A three-view (left lateral, right lateral, and ventrodorsal/dorsoventral) radiographic study of the thorax should be performed, looking for evidence of pulmonary metastatic disease.

Comment: Primary bone tumors, most commonly osteosarcoma, of the distal radius can be osteoproductive, osteolytic, or a combination of the two. The periosteal proliferation associated with these lesions can be varied, as seen in this case, ranging from smooth to spiculated to amorphous in appearance. Osteosarcoma of the distal radius and proximal humerus are the two most common sites of disease. A definitive diagnosis is obtained with a fine needle aspirate, bone biopsy, or amputation of the limb. Ultrasound and/ or fluoroscopy can be used as a guide for obtaining aspirates or biopsy samples.

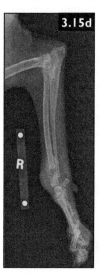

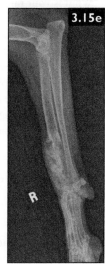

Examples of other cases of distal radial osteosarcoma are shown to demonstrate the variability in radiographic appearance of this disease (**Figs. 3.15c–e**).

Final diagnosis: Osteosarcoma.

CASE 3.16

1 What are your radiographic findings? There is a large irregular, proliferative, densely mineral opaque mass along the ventral abaxial and axial aspects of the right mandible. This mass extends from the caudal body of the right mandible dorsally along the caudal occipital bone and cranial aspect of the first cervical vertebral body. The mass also surrounds the right temporomandibular joint. Soft tissue swelling is present ventrally and laterally, adjacent to the mass.

2 What is your radiographic diagnosis? Craniomandibular osteopathy (CMO).

Comment: CMO is a self-limiting, bony proliferative disease, most commonly seen in young (3–8 months of age) Terrier breeds such as the West Highland White Terrier. The irregular osseous proliferation involves the mandible and tympanic bullae. The osseous proliferation is typically irregular in contour and bilateral, although it may be asymmetrical between the left and right sides of the head. The etiology of the disease is unknown. Discomfort often arises when the proliferation impinges on the temporomandibular joint and causes difficulties in chewing.

CASE 3.17

1 What are your radiographic findings? The right capital physis is widened with mild caudal displacement of the right femoral neck. The right femoral neck is smaller in size than the left, most consistent with resorption. The left capital physis is widened and mildly irregular in contour.

2 What is your radiographic diagnosis? Bilateral femoral capital physeal fractures.

Comment: Unilateral or bilateral femoral capital physeal fractures are common in cats, specifically obese males, and can be idiopathic or associated with trauma. In cats, the femoral capital physis typically closes between 30 and 40 weeks of age and fracture of the physis most commonly occurs between 4 and 11 months of age. On radiographs, the femoral capital physis can be just mildly widened to completely displaced. Depending on the duration of clinical signs, osteolysis and/or sclerosis of the femoral neck may also be evident. Ventrodorsal views of the pelvis, including a ventrodorsal flexed view (frog-leg view), are the most helpful in identifying the fractures.

Final diagnosis: Idiopathic femoral capital physeal fractures.

CASE 3.18

1 What are your radiographic findings? The femoral head is subluxated from the acetabulum, bilaterally. The left and right acetabula are shallow, with sclerosis of the subchondral bone. Osteophytes are present along the cranial acetabular margins, bilaterally. Both femoral heads are misshapen. Osteophytes are present along the thickened left and right femoral necks.

2 What is your radiographic diagnosis? Bilateral hip dysplasia with secondary osteoarthritis.

Comment: Compared with Case 3.6, this dog has bilateral disease with more advanced osteoarthritis. With bilateral disease, muscle atrophy may be difficult to appreciate if the musculature is still symmetrical between the left and right limbs.
   Final diagnosis: Hip dysplasia, bilateral.

CASE 3.19

1 What are your radiographic findings? A large, well-mineralized osseous body, with mildly irregular margins, is present along the caudomedial aspect of the right elbow joint. A moderately sized concave defect is present in the adjacent medial humeral epicondyle, with a moderate amount of mildly irregular osseous proliferation. A mild amount of soft tissue swelling is present along the medial elbow.

2 What is your radiographic diagnosis? Avulsion fracture of the right medial humeral epicondyle.

Comment: The tendons responsible for flexion of the carpus and phalanges originate from the medial epicondyle of the distal humerus. These tendons include the deep digital flexor tendon, superficial flexor tendon, flexor carpi ulnaris, flexor carpi radialis, and the pronator teres. An avulsion fracture of the medial humeral epicondyle is usually the result of trauma to the limb, which can occur in both young and old dogs.
   The medial epicondyle forms from a separate ossification center in the distal humerus and fuses to the distal humeral physis at approximately 10 weeks of age in the dog.
   Earlier reports have suggested that this lesion in young dogs is the result of a failure of the medial epicondyle ossification center to fuse to the distal humeral physis or is a form of osteochondrosis, as some lesions are present bilaterally in dogs without a history of trauma.

CASE 3.20

1 What are your radiographic findings? A long oblique, mid-diaphyseal fracture is present in the right humerus. The fracture is oriented in a proximomedial to distolateral direction with mild proximal and medial displacement.

Marked amorphous periosteal proliferation is present along the cranial and lateral margins of the humerus. Additionally, mildly irregular to laminar periosteal proliferation is present along the caudal and medial humeral diaphysis. The cranial and lateral cortices of the humerus are thin. A marked amount of soft tissue swelling is present surrounding the proximal right humerus.

2 What is your radiographic diagnosis? Aggressive, primarily proliferative, lesion of the proximal right humerus with a long oblique, diaphyseal pathologic fracture. The primary differential diagnosis is neoplasia.

3 Are additional radiographic views needed? A three-view (left lateral, right lateral, and ventrodorsal/dorsoventral) radiographic study of the thorax should be performed, looking for evidence of pulmonary metastatic disease.

Comment: Osteosarcoma is, by far, the most common osseous neoplasia in the proximal humerus, followed by fibrosarcoma, chondrosarcoma, and hemangiosarcoma. Primary osseous neoplasia of the humerus is most commonly identified within the proximal humeral metaphysis. The lesions are typically osteolytic, osteoproliferative, or a combination of lysis and proliferation. A fine needle aspirate or biopsy of the bone could be obtained to obtain a more definitive diagnosis.

These radiographs of proximal humeral osteosarcomas show the variability in appearance of these lesions (**Figs. 3.20c–e**).

Final diagnosis: Hemangiosarcoma.

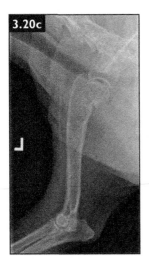
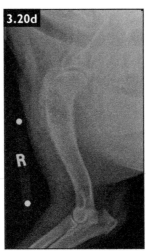
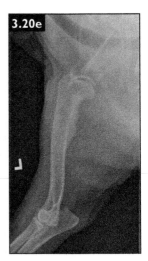

CASE 3.21

1 What are your radiographic findings? A cranially displaced oblique fracture is present through the caudoventral body of the 7th lumbar vertebral body. The fracture is oriented in a caudodorsal to cranioventral direction. Note how the fracture margins are not very sharp and a mild amount of bony callus is present along the ventral aspect of the caudal fracture fragment, consistent with a more chronic fracture and early attempts at healing. Additionally, the sacrum is cranioventrally displaced with respect to

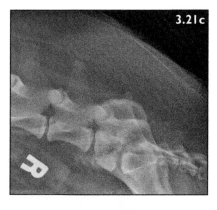

the cranial L7 vertebral fragment, with luxation of the lumbosacral articular facets.

2 What is your radiographic diagnosis? Fracture of the 7th lumbar vertebral body.

3 Are additional radiographic views needed? A view of the caudal lumbar spine, collimated over the L7 vertebral body, would be helpful (**Fig. 3.21c**).

Comment: This fracture is difficult to visualize on the ventrodorsal view as the fracture is not displaced laterally. Therefore, this case is a good example of why at least two orthogonal projections need to be performed in every radiographic examination to minimize lesions being missed.

Final diagnosis: Vertebral body fracture, L7.

CASE 3.22

1 What are your radiographic findings? The medial aspect of the coronoid process of the proximal ulna has an abnormal elongated, sharply marginated contour on the craniocaudal view and is indistinct on the lateral view. A moderate amount of soft tissue swelling is present within the elbow joint, consistent with effusion/synovial proliferation; however, no degenerative changes of the joint are identified. A cone-shaped lucency is present in the distal metaphysis of the ulna (**Fig. 3.22b**), consistent with a retained cartilaginous core. The distal metaphyses of the radius and ulna are flared and sclerotic. Ill-defined lucencies are present in the metaphyseal bone of the distal radius. Additionally, the radius and ulna are bowed cranially (radius curvus). Also of note, small, thin mineral opaque lines are present in a transverse orientation across the mid-diaphysis of the radius on the lateral view, consistent with growth arrest lines. On the carpal views, there is lateral deviation of the distal extremity, centered on the carpus.

231

2 What is your radiographic diagnosis? Left elbow dysplasia (medial coronoid disease) with effusion/synovial proliferation; hypertrophic osteodystrophy (HOD) of the left distal radius and ulna; retained cartilaginous core of the left distal ulna; left valgus angular limb deformity, centered on the carpus.

3 Are additional radiographic views needed? Radiographs of the contralateral limb would be recommended as elbow dysplasia and HOD are commonly bilateral. Lateral and craniocaudal views of the right antebrachium are shown (**Figs. 3.22e, f**), with radiographic changes very similar to the left forelimb.

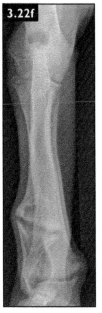

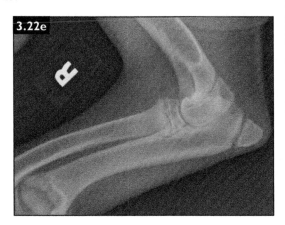

Comment: Canine elbow dysplasia is a term used to describe a group of developmental disorders that occur in the elbow, and any one or all may be present for a diagnosis of elbow dysplasia to be made. These disorders include medial coronoid disease (with or without fragmentation), ununited or fractured anconeal process, distal humeral osteochondrosis, and elbow incongruity. All of these conditions eventually lead to elbow osteoarthritis. Elbow dysplasia typically occurs in large breed dogs that are rapidly growing and is usually bilateral. The radiographic projections used to make the diagnosis include lateromedial, craniocaudal, and flexed lateromedial projections. The lateromedial view is used for evaluation of the medial aspect of the coronoid process, joint congruity, and the anconeal process. The craniocaudal projection allows for better assessment of the medial aspect of the coronoid process; however, in some dogs this view may have to be mildly obliqued in a lateromedial direction for the best visualization. The flexed lateromedial view moves the medial epicondyle of the distal humerus away from the ulna and gives the best view of the anconeal process, to detect any evidence of separation or early osteophyte formation proximally.

HOD also commonly affects large, young rapidly growing dogs. The etiology of the disease is unknown, although many potential causes, such as canine distemper virus infection, oversupplementation, and genetics, have been proposed. Lesions are typically bilateral and most commonly in the distal radius, ulna, and tibia. Radiographically, lesions of HOD are present in the metaphyseal region of long bones and include radiolucent lines parallel to the physis ('double physeal line'), sclerosis, flaring, and periosteal proliferation. Additionally, the distal physis may be irregular and widened.

Similar to the conditions discussed above, retained cartilaginous cores of the ulna are most commonly identified in large, rapidly growing dogs. They form as a result of abnormal endochondral ossification and lead to premature ceasing of ulnar growth. As the radius continues to grow, the rate of growth between the radius and ulna is no longer synchronous and this leads to incongruity of the elbow, a cranial bowing in the diaphysis of the radius, and valgus angular limb deformities of the distal limb. The diagnosis is made radiographically by visualization of a triangular lucency in the metaphysis of the distal ulna.

CASE 3.23

1 What are your radiographic findings? Increased soft tissue opacity is present within the tibiotarsal joint, consistent with effusion and/or synovial proliferation. The medial trochlear ridge of the talus is flattened on both views with widening of the medial tarsocrural joint space on the dorsoplantar view. The adjacent medial tibial subchondral bone is sclerotic. A mild to moderate amount of periarticular osteophyte formation is present circumferentially along the distal tibia and medial aspect of the talus. Smoothly marginated periosteal proliferation is also present along the cranial distal aspect of the tibia. A moderately sized well-mineralized osteochondral fragment is present in the plantar aspect of the tibiotarsal joint on the lateral view.

2 What is your radiographic diagnosis? Osteochondrosis of the right medial trochlear ridge of the talus and secondary tarsocrural osteoarthritis.

3 Are additional radiographs needed? Radiographs of the contralateral limb would be recommended as osteochondrosis is typically a bilateral condition.

Comment: Osteochondrosis most commonly occurs in young, rapidly growing large breed dogs. When a flap of cartilage is formed or osteochondral fragments are present, the lesion is referred to as osteochondritis dissecans (OCD). Most cases of tarsal osteochondrosis involve the plantar aspect of the medial trochlear ridge of the talus. Osteochondrosis lesions of the lateral trochlear ridge are also identified, most commonly in the Rottweiler breed. Standard lateromedial and dorsoplantar radiographic views are typically obtained first, and then flexed lateral and oblique

233

views can be made to aid in making the diagnosis. Radiographic abnormalities indicative of osteochondrosis include increased soft tissue opacity within the tibiotarsal joint, flattening of the trochlear ridge, widening of the joint space, and possibly osteochondral fragments within the joint. If osteochondrosis lesions are left untreated, secondary osteoarthritis will likely develop.

Computed tomography (CT) can be used to confirm the radiographic diagnosis and define the location of any fragments that may be present. CT images from a dog with medial trochlear ridge osteochondrosis are shown (**Figs. 3.23c, d**).

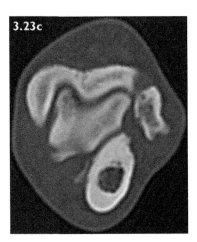

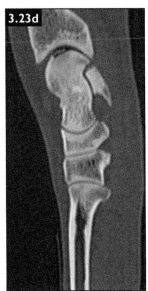

CASE 3.24

1 What are your radiographic findings? A moderate increase in soft tissue opacity is present within the stifle joint, with effacement of the infrapatellar fat pad, consistent with effusion and/or synovial proliferation. There is also thickening of the soft tissues along the medial aspect of the stifle joint, known as a 'medial buttress'. Small smoothly marginated osteophytes are present on the proximal femoral trochlea, medial and lateral femoral epicondyles, apex of the patella, medial fabella, and medial and lateral aspects of the tibial condyles. Note also the steep angle of the caudal tibial plateau on the lateral view.

2 What is your radiographic diagnosis? Moderate left stifle effusion and/or synovial proliferation with mild osteoarthritis. These findings are most likely associated with ligamentous instability, such as a tear in the cranial cruciate ligament.

Comment: Cranial cruciate injuries are the most common cause of ligamentous instability in the canine stifle. Increased soft tissue opacity within the joint, likely associated with effusion, is typically the first radiographic change visualized after injury to the cranial crucial ligament. Osteophytes can be identified on radiographs within about 2 weeks after injury. Osteophytes within the stifle are commonly seen along the femoral trochlea, patella, fabellae, and proximal tibial condyles. The medial buttress effect is the result of thickening of the medial collateral ligament of the stifle joint and can be palpated clinically. Some have hypothesized that a steep caudal angle of the proximal tibial plateau could predispose dogs to damage of the cranial cruciate ligament; however, steep angles have been measured in clinically normal dogs and dogs with cranial cruciate ligament rupture.

Final diagnosis: Cranial cruciate ligament rupture.

CASE 3.25

1 What are your radiographic findings? A marked amount of irregular to amorphous osseous proliferation is present surrounding the right elbow joint and adjacent soft tissues. The distal humerus and proximal radius and ulna are heterogeneous in opacity with multiple areas of osteolysis. The osteolytic regions extend into the subchondral bone and to the articular surfaces. The elbow joint space is also markedly narrowed. Marked soft tissue swelling is present surrounding the elbow and proximal antebrachium.

2 What is your radiographic diagnosis? Aggressive, markedly osteoproductive and osteolytic lesion of the right elbow, most consistent with neoplasia.

3 Are additional radiographs needed? A three-view radiographic study of the thorax would be recommended, looking for evidence of metastasis.

Comment: Synovial neoplasia is relatively uncommon in veterinary patients. The most common synovial tumor in dogs and cats is synovial cell sarcoma, which usually occurs in the stifle and elbow joints. A fine needle aspirate or biopsy of the elbow joint lesion would need to be obtained to determine a definitive diagnosis.

Final diagnosis: Osteosarcoma.

CASE 3.26

1 What are your radiographic findings? The right radial head is caudally and laterally luxated from the articulation with the distal humerus. The radial diaphysis is bowed cranially and medially. The proximal ulnar diaphysis is angled caudally. Increased soft tissue opacity is present within the cranial and caudal aspects of elbow joint and surrounding the elbow and proximal antebrachium.

2 What is your radiographic diagnosis? Caudolateral luxation of the proximal right radius.

Comment: Elbow luxations are the result of displacement of the proximal radius and/or ulna from the articulation with the distal humerus and can be due to trauma or congenital defects. The luxation is more commonly in a lateral direction due to the larger medial condyle of the distal humerus. Radiographs are used to confirm the diagnosis.
   Final diagnosis: Congenital elbow luxation.

CASE 3.27
1 What are your radiographic findings? The proximal femoral physes are mildly widened and irregular in contour, best visualized on the flexed ventrodorsal view. No evidence of secondary degenerative joint disease is present.
2 What is your radiographic diagnosis? Bilateral capital physeal femoral fractures.

Comment: The proximal femoral physis closes in dogs between 6 and 9 months of age; however, in some canine patients this physis has been reported remain open until almost 12 months of age. Femoral capital physeal fractures can be unilateral or bilateral and are typically best visualized on the neutral or flexed ventrodorsal (frog-leg) projection. Radiographic signs of a capital physeal fracture range from widening or irregularity of the physis to complete displacement of the fracture. Coxofemoral osteoarthritis and subluxation are common sequelae to these fractures.

CASE 3.28
1 What are your radiographic findings? The intervertebral disk space at the lumbosacral junction is collapsed. A moderate amount of sclerosis is present along the caudal L7 and cranial S1 endplates; however, no endplate lysis is present. Ventrally and laterally, smoothly marginated spondylosis deformans is present at the level of the lumbosacral space. The pelvis, coxofemoral joints, and proximal femurs are unremarkable.
2 What is your radiographic diagnosis? Marked lumbosacral degeneration.

Comment: Degenerative lumbosacral disease is common in older, large breed dogs and is believed to be the result of disk degeneration and instability at the lumbosacral junction. Radiographic signs of lumbosacral disease include narrowing of the intervertebral disk space, spondylosis deformans, sclerosis of the caudal L7 and cranial S1 endplates, articular facet proliferation, and stenosis of

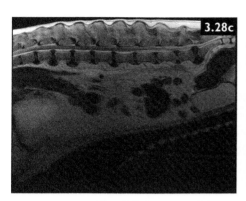

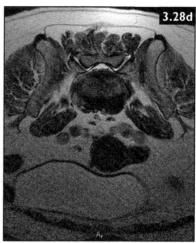

the vertebral canal. As the disease progresses, the protrusion of the intervertebral disk into the ventral vertebral canal, osseous proliferation, and hypertrophy of the interarcuate ligament may cause impingement of the nerve roots in the caudal vertebral canal or as they exit through the intervertebral foramina. Myelography, computed tomography and magnetic resonance imaging (MRI) have been used to evaluate the extent of lumbosacral intervertebral disk protrusion and associated osseous changes.

T2 sagittal (**Fig. 3.28c**) and T2 axial (**Fig. 3.28d**) MR images of a dog with lumbosacral degeneration and protrusion of the intervertebral disk are shown.

CASE 3.29

1 What are your radiographic findings? A large, well-mineralized, irregularly contoured anconeal process fragment is present and separated by a wide area of lucency from the ulnar diaphysis. This separation is accentuated on the flexed lateral view. There is moderate sclerosis along the trochlear notch of the ulna. The medial aspect of the coronoid process of the ulna is blunted and proliferative on the craniocaudal view and indistinct on the lateral view. Osteophytes are present along the medial epicondyle of the distal humerus and cranioproximal radius. Increased soft tissue opacity is present within the elbow joint, consistent with effusion and/or synovial proliferation.

2 What is your radiographic diagnosis? Right elbow dysplasia with a fractured or ununited anconeal process and medial coronoid disease; mild right elbow osteoarthritis.

3 Are additional radiographs needed? Radiographs of the left elbow would be recommended as elbow dysplasia is commonly a bilateral condition. These radiographs of the left elbow (**Figs. 3.29d–f**) show very similar findings to those described for the right elbow.

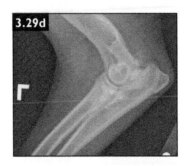

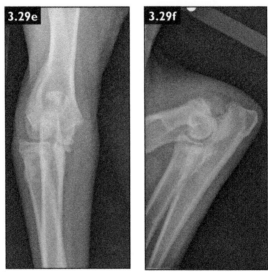

Comment: In puppies of medium and large breeds, a very small, poorly defined separate center of ossification of the anconeal process of the ulna has been identified. This separate center of ossification is typically more cranial in location than the irregular separation seen with an ununited or fractured anconeal process. Additionally, this separate ossification center is usually smaller in size than the large anconeal process fracture fragments. In most dogs, the anconeal process center of ossification fuses to the ulnar diaphysis by 5 months of age.

Final diagnosis: Bilateral elbow dysplasia.

CASE 3.30

1 What are your radiographic findings? The lateral femoral condyle is flattened with sclerosis of the subchondral bone, best visualized on the lateral view. No effusion or degenerative changes of the stifle joint are identified.

2 What is your radiographic diagnosis? Left lateral femoral condyle osteochondrosis.

3 Are additional radiographs needed? Radiographs of the right stifle should be performed as osteochondrosis is typically a bilaterally condition.

Comment: Osteochondrosis lesions of the canine stifle joint occur most commonly along the axial aspect of the lateral femoral condyle; however, lesions have also been reported along the medial femoral condyle. Radiographic signs of the stifle joint include a flattening or concavity in the subchondral bone of the distal femur with adjacent sclerosis. Do not mistake the extensor fossa, a normal concavity along the abaxial aspect of the lateral femoral condyle, for an osteochondrosis lesion.

Lateromedial and caudocranial images of a normal stifle with the extensor fossa highlighted are shown

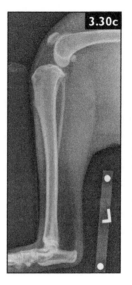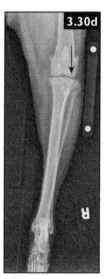

(**Figs. 3.30c, d**). Also note the normal amount of soft tissue opacity within the stifle joint and large, normal infrapatellar fat pad.

CASE 3.31

1 What are your radiographic findings? There is an oblique fracture of the second phalanx of the fourth digit, with proximal, medial, and palmar displacement. The fracture also has palmar angulation on the lateral view. The soft tissues of the fourth digit, from the distal metacarpus to the distal phalanx, are swollen.

2 What is your radiographic diagnosis? Oblique fracture of the second phalanx of the left fourth digit.

Comment: If a lesion of the phalanges is suspected, a lateral view with the digits spread apart is recommended. Tape works well to separate the toes and is usually well tolerated by the patient. If soft tissue swelling is present, but a lesion is not identified, additional oblique views could be performed to ensure a nondisplaced fracture is not present.

CASE 3.32

1 What are your radiographic findings? A marked increase in soft tissue opacity is present within the cranial and caudal aspects of the stifle joint, with effacement of the infrapatellar fat pad, consistent with effusion and/or synovial proliferation. On the lateral view, two small sharply marginated osseous fragments are present in the cranial stifle joint and adjacent to an ill-defined lucency in the cranioproximal tibia, near the insertion of the cranial cruciate ligament. These fragments can also be visualized on the caudocranial view, medial to the intercondylar eminence of the proximal tibia. No degenerative changes of the stifle joint are identified.

2 What is your radiographic diagnosis? Left proximal tibial avulsion fracture of the insertion of the cranial cruciate ligament with marked stifle effusion/synovial proliferation.

Comment: The cranial cruciate ligament originates from the lateral portion of the intercondylar fossa (axial portion of the lateral femoral condyle) and inserts along the cranial aspect of the proximal tibial plateau. Damage to the cranial cruciate ligament is typically the result of stifle hyperextension. Avulsion of the insertion of the cranial cruciate has been reported more commonly than avulsion of the origin. Additionally, cranial cruciate avulsion fractures have been identified more commonly in immature dogs than in adult dogs, possibly due to the strength of the tendinous fibers compared with the strength of the bone in young dogs. In this patient, radiographs of the contralateral stifle revealed an identical lesion.

CASE 3.33

1 What are your radiographic findings? A concave lucency is present in the subchondral bone of the medial distal humeral condyle with adjacent subchondral sclerosis. The medial aspect of the coronoid process of the ulna is indistinct on the lateral view and blunted on the craniocaudal view. Smoothly marginated osseous proliferation is present along the dorsal aspect of the anconeal process. There is incongruity of the humeroradial joint.

2 What is your radiographic diagnosis? Left elbow dysplasia characterized by medial coronoid disease and distal medial humeral osteochondrosis.

3 Are additional radiographs needed? Radiographs of the contralateral limb would be recommended as elbow dysplasia is commonly bilateral.

Comment: Recheck radiographs of the left elbow taken 2 years later are shown (**Figs. 3.33c, d**). Note the progression of the osteoarthritis with an increase in osteophyte production along the medial humeral epicondyle, proximal anconeal process of the ulna, and cranioproximal radius. Also note the increase in proliferation along the medial aspect of the coronoid process of the ulna.

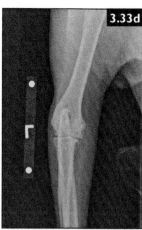

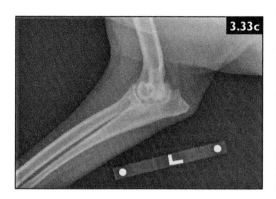

CASE 3.34

1 What are your radiographic findings? There is comminuted fracture of the mid-body of the patella with marked proximal and distal displacement. The proximal fracture fragment is a single large fragment. However, the distal portion of the fracture is composed of three larger fragments and multiple very small fragments. Additionally, small mineral opacities are present at the insertion of the patellar ligament. There is swelling of the soft tissues along the cranial aspect of the stifle joint. A mild increase in soft tissue opacity is present within the stifle joint, consistent with effusion and/or synovial proliferation.

2 What is your radiographic diagnosis? Comminuted left patellar fracture.

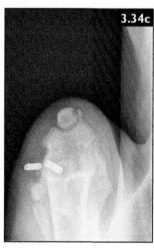

Comment: Patellar fractures have been reported in dogs and cats secondary to direct or indirect trauma. Fractures of the patella can occur in many different configurations, including transverse, sagittal, comminuted, and nondisplaced. If a patellar fracture is suspected but not demonstrated on standard lateral or craniocaudal views, a skyline view of the patella could be performed.

This skyline projection of a patellar fracture in a different patient (**Fig. 3.34c**) nicely shows how the skyline view is useful in depicting patellar fractures. The two small metallic objects are from a previous stifle stabilization surgery.

CASE 3.35

1 What are your radiographic findings? The intervertebral disk space of L2-3 is markedly narrowed. The caudal L2 and cranial L3 endplates are sclerotic and irregular in contour, with areas of endplate erosion. Spondylosis deformans is also present ventrally at L2-3. Spondylosis deformans is present at L1-2, without evidence of vertebral endplate changes or disc space narrowing.

2 What is your radiographic diagnosis? Diskospondylitis at L2-3.

3 Are additional radiographs needed? Radiographs of the entire spine should be obtained, looking for other sites of diskospondylitis and to serve as a baseline for recheck examinations.

Comment: Diskospondylitis occurs secondary to hematogenous spread of infection (e.g. urinary tract infection), iatrogenic, penetrating wounds, or migration of foreign material (e.g. grass awns). Radiographic signs of diskospondylitis include narrowing to collapse of the intervertebral disk space, osteolysis and sclerosis of the vertebral endplates, and spondylosis or new bone around the intervertebral disk space. These signs vary depending on the stage in the disease process and may not always correlate with clinical signs. However, if diskospondylitis is suspected clinically and radiographs do not demonstrate a lesion, repeat radiographs in 7–10 days would be recommended. Additionally, magnetic resonance imaging (MRI) can be used to identify diskospondylitis and may be more sensitive for detecting early disease when compared with radiographs.

T2 sagittal (**Fig. 3.35c**) and STIR coronal (**Fig. 3.35d**) MR images of a patient with discospondylitis at L3-4 and L4-5 are shown. Note the hyperintense vertebral endplates on the STIR image. Additional signs of diskospondylitis on MRI include intervertebral disk space narrowing and irregular margination, hyperintense and contrast-enhancing vertebral endplates, and variable hyperintensity and contrast enhancement of the adjacent paravertebral musculature.

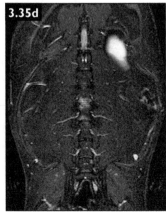

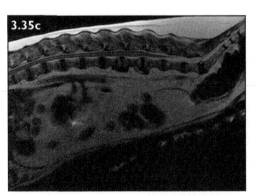

CASE 3.36

1 What are your radiographic findings? A large, expansile, osteolytic lesion is present within the proximal to mid-diaphysis of the right tibia. Sclerosis and irregular periosteal reaction extends from the proximal to the distal diaphysis of the right tibia. Moderate soft tissue swelling surrounds the right tibia.

2 What is your radiographic diagnosis? Aggressive, osteolytic right tibial mid-diaphyseal lesion. The primary differential diagnoses include osteomyelitis and metastatic neoplasia.

Comment: Osteomyelitis and neoplasia can be difficult to distinguish on radiographs, therefore a fine needle aspirate or biopsy (+/– culture) of the bone would be recommended for a definitive diagnosis. Osteomyelitis in the dog can be caused by bacterial (most commonly *Staphylococcus* species), fungal, or viral organisms. Osteomyelitis is the result of direct contamination of the bone (e.g. wounds, surgery, open fractures, foreign body migration), extension from a soft tissue infection, or hematogenous spread (e.g. urinary tract infection). Bone is relatively good at resisting infection; however, these defenses are compromised when the bone is damaged, such as after a traumatic event or surgery. Common radiographic signs of osteomyelitis are soft tissue swelling, periosteal proliferation, and osteolysis. Osteomyelitis can occur in any location; however, in young animals it is more common in the metaphyseal region of long bones. One or multiple bones can be affected. If a draining tract is present, a fistulogram (placement of sterile iodinated contrast within the tract) could be performed using radiography or computed tomography to confirm extension of the tract to the bone.

Final diagnosis: Bacterial osteomyelitis.

CASE 3.37

1 What are your radiographic findings? Sharply marginated transverse fractures are present through the mid-diaphysis of the right radius and ulna. The fractures are proximally and laterally displaced with caudal angulation. Small fissures extend proximally for approximately 2.5 cm within the radial diaphysis. A small osseous fragment is present along the caudolateral aspect of the distal ulnar fracture fragment. Gas is present in the soft tissues cranial and medial to the fracture. A marked amount of soft tissue swelling is present surrounding the antebrachium. Incidentally, smoothly marginated osteophytes are present along the cranioproximal radius. The medial coronoid process of the right ulna is blunted and proliferative.

2 What is your radiographic diagnosis? Diaphyseal, displaced transverse open fractures of the right radius and ulna.

Comment: Fractures are described by location (metaphyseal, diaphyseal, epiphyseal, physeal, articular), orientation (transverse, spiral, oblique), and number of fracture fragments (simple vs. comminuted). Additional descriptors used to describe fractures include the following: open vs. closed, complete vs. incomplete, and occasionally words to describe the type of pathology/injury (compression, shearing, fissure, osteochondral, chip, or avulsion). Displacement of the fracture is described relative to the distal or caudal fracture fragment. Incomplete or nondisplaced fractures can sometimes be difficult to detect on initial radiographs. If a fracture is suspected but not identified on the initial orthogonal projections, oblique radiographic views of the area, computed tomography, or nuclear scintigraphy could be performed. Alternatively, repeat radiographs in 7–10 days may reveal remodeling of the fracture and/or early periosteal proliferation that was not immediately evident after an acute injury.

CASE 3.38

1 What are your radiographic findings? Marked spondylosis deformans is present laterally and ventrally from T12 to the sacrum. The spondylosis is more severe on the left at T12-13, L5-6, L6-7, and L7-S1. A mild amount of linear mineral opacity is present along the dorsal aspect of the intervertebral disk spaces throughout the lumbar spine, which may be mineralization of the annulus fibrosis or superimposed lateralized spondylosis. The articular facets of the L3-4 and L4-5 articulations are proliferative, consistent with osteoarthritis.

2 What is your radiographic diagnosis? Marked degenerative spinal changes throughout the caudal thoracic and lumbar spine, marked diffuse spondylosis, and mid-lumbar articular facet osteoarthrosis.

Comment: Spondylosis deformans is a noninflammatory bony reaction along the intervertebral spaces. It is typically smooth and ranges in size from small osteophytes to complete bridges of bone between vertebral bodies. Spondylosis commonly affects the thoracic and lumbar spine in older dogs and may or may not be present at sites of intervertebral disk narrowing. Spondylosis is usually an incidental finding; however, if the bony proliferation is severe or forms dorsally, it can cause impingement on the nerve roots and irritation of the meninges.

CASE 3.39

1 What are your radiographic findings? There is a mild increase in soft tissue opacity within the left nasal cavity with loss of the normal nasal turbinate architecture. The nasal septum is within normal limits, with no evidence of a mass effect.

2 What is your radiographic diagnosis? Unilateral aggressive, osteolytic nasal disease (left-sided). The primary differential diagnoses for destructive/aggressive nasal disease include: fungal rhinitis or neoplasia.

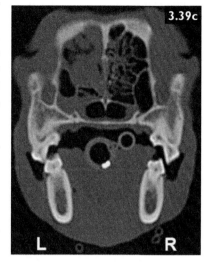

3.39c

3 Is additional imaging needed? Computed tomography (CT) or magnetic resonance imaging (MRI) of the skull could be performed to further evaluate the degree of osteolysis and turbinate destruction, determine if the soft tissue opacity is vascularized tissue in comparison with mucus/fluid/debris, and identify if any extension through the cribriform plate into the brain is present.

Comment: CT is more commonly used for nasal diseases, in comparison with MRI, as bone margins are better delineated and the examination is often faster. An axial CT image from this patient is shown (**Fig. 3.39c**).

Final diagnosis: Destructive rhinitis secondary to aspergillosis.

CASE 3.40

1 What are your radiographic findings? The right femoral head is misshapen and flattened cranially with moderate thickening of the right femoral neck and a mild to moderate amount of smoothly marginated osseous proliferation on the femoral neck adjacent to this flattening. There is a moderate amount of osteophyte formation on the cranial aspect of the right acetabular rim and the right femoral head is subluxated. There is a marked decrease in soft tissue of the right gluteal musculature and surrounding the right proximal hindlimb.

2 What is your radiographic diagnosis? Severely misshapen right femoral head with secondary degenerative joint disease and severe muscle atrophy. The most likely diagnosis is avascular necrosis of the femoral head (Legg–Calvé–Perthes disease).

Comment: This disease is commonly seen in small and toy breeds. It may be unilateral or bilateral. Femoral head excision ostectomy is curative. This example shows long-standing pathology. Many cases present with lameness early in the disease process and thus the radiographic findings can be subtle.

Final diagnosis: Avascular necrosis of the femoral head.

CASE 3.41

1 What are your radiographic findings? There is moderate subluxation of the middle carpal joint with caudal displacement of the distal row of carpal bones with respect to the proximal row of carpal bones. An osteochondral fragment is present dorsally at the level of the distal row of carpal bones. A fragment is also present along the palmar distal ulnar carpal bone. On the stressed view, there is excessive extension of the carpus (>40 degrees). The accessory carpal bone has an abnormal angulation, consistent with damage to the palmar ligaments.

2 What is your radiographic diagnosis? Caudal subluxation of the right middle carpal bone and small fractures of the dorsodistal carpus and palmar ulnar carpal bone, consistent with a hyperextension injury.

Comment: Hyperextension injuries can occur in the dog after an acute traumatic event or repetitive injury that causes damage to the palmar support for the carpus, which includes the palmar carpal ligaments and fibrocartilage. These injuries are most common in older, large breed dogs. On initial radiographs, effusion is the most common finding. Small fracture fragments along the dorsal aspect of the joint may be also visualized following a traumatic event. Signs of osteoarthritis (osteophytes, enthesophytes, joint narrowing, and/or subluxation) will be seen after chronic or repetitive injury. A stressed lateromedial view of the carpus is commonly performed to confirm hyperextension.

   Final diagnosis: Carpal hyperextension injury.

CASE 3.42

1 What are your radiographic findings? The supraglenoid tubercle of the distal scapula is fractured with distal displacement of the fracture fragment as illustrated on the flexed lateral projection (**Fig. 3.42c**). The fracture margins are mildly indistinct. The remainder of the shoulder is within normal limits.

2 What is your radiographic diagnosis? Right supraglenoid tubercle fracture.

Comment: Fractures of the supraglenoid tubercle occur most commonly in young dogs as the tubercle has a separate center of ossification. This separate center of ossification fuses by approximately 3–5 months of age. Additionally, the supraglenoid tubercle is the origin for the biceps brachii tendon, therefore fractures of the supraglenoid tubercle can also be associated with avulsion of the biceps tendon.

CASE 3.43

1 What are your radiographic findings? Left: the subchondral bone of the distal humerus, proximal ulna, and proximal radius is markedly irregular and erosive. Marked narrowing of the humeroradial joint is present and the humeroulnar joint is severely incongruent. Marked osteophyte formation is present along the medial and lateral epicondyles of the distal humerus, cranioproximal radius, and proximal anconeal process of the ulna. Additionally, the proximal ulnar diaphysis is sclerotic and mottled in opacity. The olecranon fossa of the distal humerus is enlarged and irregularly marginated. Marked soft tissue swelling is present surrounding the elbow.

Right: the findings in the right elbow are almost identical to the left.

2 What is your radiographic diagnosis? Severe bilateral erosive arthritis of the elbows.

Comment: Differentials for polyarticular erosive arthritis include infection (bacteremia), systemic inflammation (e.g. leishmaniasis, Lyme disease, *Mycoplasma*), and immune-mediated joint disease (e.g. rheumatoid arthritis). Radiographically, increased soft tissue opacity in the joint (effusion and/or synovial hyperplasia) is a common finding and may be the only abnormality early in the course of disease. Osteophyte formation, sclerosis, and erosions of the subchondral bone and narrowing to collapse of the joint space can also be identified on radiographs as the disease progresses. Cytologic analysis and culture of the joint fluid is used to determine a more definitive diagnosis.

Final diagnosis: Immune-mediated erosive polyarthropathy.

CASE 3.44

1 What are your radiographic findings? A large, well-defined, smoothly marginated mineral opaque mass is present within the occipital region of the skull. This mineral opacity extends ventral to the dorsal aspect of the calvarium on the lateral view, consistent with intracranial extension.

2 What is your radiographic diagnosis? Large intracranial mineralized occipital mass. The most likely diagnosis is a multilobular tumor (MLO) of bone.

3 Is additional imaging needed? Magnetic resonance imaging (MRI) or computed tomography (CT) of the skull is used to determine the extent of intracranial extension and subsequent compression of the brain. A T2 sagittal MR image of the skull of this patient shows the marked caudal cerebral and cerebellar compression by the mass (**Fig. 3.44c**).

3.44c

Comment: MLO is a tumor of the cranium that commonly originates from the temporal/occipital bones and is most often seen in older, large breed dogs. This tumor is also known as multilobular osteochondrosarcoma, chondroma rodens, and multilobular osteoma. On radiographs, these lesions are well-defined, primarily proliferative

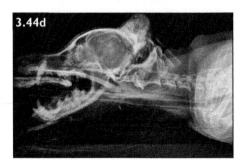

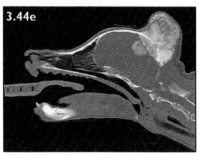

masses composed of coarse to finely granular mineral opacity. A radiograph (**Fig. 3.44d**) and a sagittal CT scan (**Fig. 3.44e**) from another patient with an MLO of bone are shown. Note how coarsely textured this mass is in comparison with the example above.

CASE 3.45

1 What are your radiographic findings? A large irregularly marginated osseous fragment is adjacent to an undulating, concave defect in the proximomedial margin of the calcaneal tuber. This osseous fragment is within an enlarged common calcaneal tendinous insertion. On the lateral view, the proximal plantar aspect of the calcaneus has a mild amount of smoothly marginated proliferation with a sharply marginated protuberance pointing ventrally. Osteophytes are present along the dorsal aspect of the distal intertarsal joint.

2 What is your radiographic diagnosis? Avulsion fracture of the right calcaneal tuber and common calcaneal tendonopathy; right distal intertarsal joint osteoarthrosis.

3 Is additional imaging needed? Ultrasound can be used to further evaluate the degree of damage to the calcaneal tendon.

Comment: The common calcaneal tendon is composed of tendinous fibers from the gastrocnemius and superficial digital flexor tendons and muscles of the biceps femoris, gracilis, and semitendinosus and inserts on the proximal aspect of the calcaneus. Middle aged, active large breed dogs are most commonly affected with calcaneal tendonopathy. Damage to the tendon usually occurs acutely secondary to trauma or chronically due to degeneration of the tendon. On radiographs, the calcaneal tendon is easy to identify and, in cases of tendonopathy, is enlarged, which is easiest to appreciate on a lateral view. Mineralization adjacent to the proximal calcaneus may be associated with avulsion fractures or dystrophic mineralization within the tendon. In this patient, an avulsion fracture was suspected due to the concavity in the contour of the proximal calcaneus.

CASE 3.46

1 What are your radiographic findings? A large soft tissue opaque mass is present along the lateral, cranial, and caudal aspects of the proximal antebrachium, extending from the distal humerus to the mid-radius and ulna. No bony reaction or osteolysis is present adjacent to the mass. A small smoothly marginated osteophyte is present on the proximal anconeal process. On the lateral view, the medial aspect of the coronoid process is ill-defined.

2 What is your radiographic diagnosis? Large soft tissue mass along the right antebrachium; minimal right elbow osteoarthrosis.

Comment: Soft tissue masses, such as lipomas, soft tissue sarcomas, hemangiosarcomas, and mast cell tumors, are commonly encountered on the limbs. If a soft tissue mass is identified on radiographs, the images should be carefully evaluated for any evidence of bony involvement, such as osteolysis or periosteal proliferation. Also of note, this mass is composed of fat, yet looks soft tissue opaque on the radiographs, likely due to the thickness of the mass.

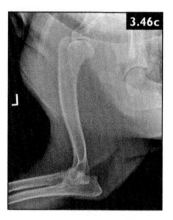

An example of another palpable soft tissue mass adjacent to the humerus is shown (**Fig. 3.46c**). On this image, however, there is evidence of bony involvement with wispy, mildly irregular periosteal proliferation along the proximal humerus.

Final diagnosis: Lipoma.

CASE 3.47

1 What are your radiographic findings? Marked soft tissue swelling is identified around the mid- to distal tibia. An indentation is identified circumferentially within this soft tissue swelling at the level of the distal tibial diaphysis. Also at this level, a circumferential rim of osteolysis is identified within the underlying tibial cortex, with flaring of the margins of this lesion. Additionally, smooth periosteal proliferation and sclerosis are identified adjacent to this osseous lesion in the tibia.

2 What is your radiographic diagnosis? Ring-like osteolysis secondary to vascular compromise and necrosis with surrounding bony reaction and severe soft tissue swelling.

Comment: Close examination following radiography showed an embedded rubber band surrounding the distal tibia, with underlying tissue necrosis. The rubber band had apparently been maliciously placed. The patient made a full recovery following débridement and management of an open wound.

CASE 3.48

1 What are your radiographic findings? The L1-2 intervertebral disk space and articular facet joint space are markedly narrowed. Ventral and lateral spondylosis deformans is also present at the L1-2 intervertebral disk space. A small mineral opacity is superimposed over the ventral aspect of the L1-2 intervertebral foramen, most consistent with extruded intervertebral disk material. The T13-L1 and L2-3 intervertebral disk spaces are also mildly narrowed with mild spondylosis. The remainder of the spine is within normal limits.

2 What is your radiographic diagnosis? Marked L1-2 intervertebral disk space narrowing with adjacent mineralization within the vertebral canal; milder T13-L1 and L1-2 intervertebral disk space narrowing, consistent with intervertebral disk disease.

Comment: The site of intervertebral disk protrusion or extrusion is difficult to definitively identify with plain radiographs. Radiographic signs of intervertebral disk disease include narrowing of the intervertebral disk space, narrowing of the articular facet joint, mineralization of the intervertebral disk, and possibly mineralized disc material within the intervertebral foramen or vertebral canal. Further imaging, such as myelography, computed tomography (CT), or magnetic resonance imaging (MRI), is commonly required to determine the exact site and location of disk protrusion/extrusion. Myelography is relatively quick and can identify the site of disk extrusion; however, the findings with myelography are not always clear, especially if artifacts due to a poor injection are present. Additionally, seizures are a potential risk of injection of iodinated contrast into the subarachnoid space for myelography. CT allows for a tomographic view of the spine and is quick and accurate for identifying sites of disk protrusion/extrusion, especially if the disk material is mineralized. The advantage of MRI over CT or myelography is the ability to assess the soft tissue structures, such as the spinal cord, for any abnormalities. On MR images, the spinal cord is commonly hyperintense on T2 images near the site of protrusion/extrusion of the disk, likely due to edema, gliosis, or hemorrhage secondary to the compression. MRI, however, does typically take longer than CT or myelography, increasing the time the patient is under general anesthesia.

T2 sagittal (**Fig. 3.48g**) and T2 axial (**Fig. 3.48h**) MR images of this patient are shown.

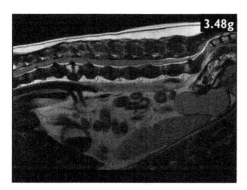

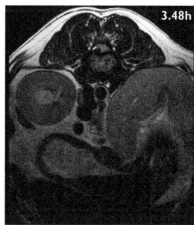

CASE 3.49

1 What are your radiographic findings? The left sacroiliac joint is cranially luxated. A sagittal fracture is present through the left ischium, extending from the caudal obturator foramen to the axial aspect of the ischial tuberosity. An oblique fracture is present through the right iliac body that extends caudally to the right acetabulum. The right femoral head is still positioned within the right acetabulum, which is axially displaced. A segmental fracture of the right acetabulum is present, best seen on the lateral view. Caudal to the acetabulum, the right ischium is fractured. The right pubis is also fractured and ventrally displaced, although this is difficult to see on the ventrodorsal view. Incidentally, ventral spondylosis deformans is present at the lumbosacral junction.

2 What is your radiographic diagnosis? Multiple pelvic fractures, including the right ilium, right acetabulum, right pubis, right ischium, and left ischium; left sacroiliac luxation.

3 Is additional imaging needed? Oblique views of the pelvis or a computed tomography examination may be needed to identify all the fractures present, as multiple pelvic fractures (>3) are present in this dog.

Comment: Pelvic fractures are almost always associated with trauma. Severe trauma to the pelvis can result in damage to structures within or near the pelvic inlet, most commonly the urinary bladder and/or urethra and peripheral nerves. A cystogram and/or urethrogram could be performed using iodinated contrast to determine if any tears are present in the urinary tract.

CASE 3.50

1 **What are your radiographic findings?** The dens, or odontoid process of the second cervical vertebral body, is not present. No other abnormalities are identified.
2 **What is your radiographic diagnosis?** Dens aplasia.

Comment: Dens aplasia is a developmental anomaly that predisposes dogs to atlantoaxial instability and possible subluxation. Atlantoaxial subluxation can also occur as a result of dens hypoplasia, absence of a transverse ligament, failure of the dens to unite to C2, or trauma. Atlantoaxial subluxation is most commonly seen in young, small breed dogs and these patients typically present with neck pain following a traumatic event. The instability at the atlantoaxial space can cause compression and damage to the cranial cervical spinal cord. Diagnosis is made on radiographs by identification of a widened space between the dorsal aspect of C1 and dorsal C2. A small or absent dens on radiographs is also a clue that instability is likely present. If the dens is difficult to visualize, a lateral oblique view could be performed to highlight the cranial aspect of C2 by removing the superimposition with the wings of C1. Evaluation can also be made in real-time with fluoroscopy and slow flexion of the neck; however, *extreme* caution must be taken as overflexion can result in spinal cord damage.

CASE 3.51

1 **What are your radiographic findings?** The right intercarpal and carpometacarpal joints are markedly narrowed; however, no erosion of the subchondral bone is present. A moderate increase in soft tissue opacity is present dorsally along the carpus, centered at the intercarpal joint, consistent with effusion and/or synovial proliferation. A mild amount of extra-articular soft tissue swelling is also present circumferentially along the carpus. On the left, a mild to moderate amount of soft tissue swelling is present dorsally along the carpus, also centered on the intercarpal joint. No osseous abnormalities are identified in the left carpus.
2 **What is your radiographic diagnosis?** Right intercarpal and carpometacarpal joint space collapse with effusion and/or synovial proliferation, consistent with a nonerosive arthritis; mild to moderate effusion/synovial proliferation of the intercarpal and carpometacarpal joints. Differentials include an immune-mediated arthropathy (i.e. systemic lupus erythematosus) or joint infection.

Comment: Immune-mediated arthropathies most commonly seen in dogs include rheumatoid arthritis or systemic lupus erythematosus. In patients with rheumatoid arthritis, radiographic signs include effusion, subchondral bone erosions, osteophytes, enthesophytes, subchondral sclerosis, and joint subluxation/luxation;

however, these changes will vary depending on the course of the disease. Joints commonly affected with rheumatoid arthritis are the distal joints in the extremities.

Patients with lupus have effusion in affected joints with minimal osseous changes seen on radiographs. Other systemic manifestations of lupus are often identified in the blood, kidneys, muscles, skin, central nervous system, and thorax. The most common joints affected include the carpus, tarsus, metatarsus, stifle, and elbow.

The primary difference between the radiographic changes seen with rheumatoid arthritis and systemic lupus erythematosus is the presence of subchondral erosions, which are common in rheumatoid arthritis and uncommon with lupus.

CASE 3.52

1 What are your radiographic findings? A transverse fracture is present through the mid-body of the left scapula that extends through the spine of the scapula. This fracture is laterally displaced. The proximal left humerus is within normal limits.
2 What is your radiographic diagnosis? Transverse left scapular fracture.

Comment: Fractures through the body, spine, or neck of the scapula can be difficult to appreciate on standard radiographs due to superimposition with the cranial thoracic structures, spine, and dorsal musculature. Oblique views of the scapula (as seen in Case 3.8) and craniocaudal/caudocranial views are often very helpful if a fracture is suspected. These fractures typically occur as a result of trauma, therefore the scapula should be carefully inspected with a history of a traumatic event, such as being hit by a car.

CASE 3.53

1 What are your radiographic findings? Mildly irregular bony proliferation is present along the ventral aspects of T13, L1, L2, and L3. Increased soft tissue opacity, with loss of serosal detail, is present in the left cranial quadrant of the abdomen. This opacity appears to be causing caudal deviation of the spleen. Increased, ill-defined soft tissue opacity is also present ventral to the L4–L7 vertebral bodies, in the region of the hypaxial musculature. Incidentally, both 13th ribs are hypoplastic.
2 What is your radiographic diagnosis? Lumbar spondylitis. Suspect a paralumbar abscess.

Comment: Spondylitis most commonly occurs secondary to infection. On radiographs, spondylitis is diagnosed by bony proliferation along the affected vertebral body. Common sites for spondylitis are L3 and L4, as the diaphragmatic

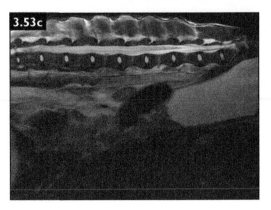
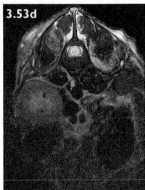

crura attach ventrally along these vertebral bodies and foreign bodies, such as plant awns, can easily migrate to these locations. Spondylitis of the thoracic vertebral bodies is also a common finding in cases of *Spirocerca lupi* infection.

T2 sagittal (**Fig. 3.53c**) and T2 axial (**Fig. 3.53d**) magnetic resonance images from this patient show marked, diffuse T2 hyperintensity throughout the lumbar spinal cord and adjacent paralumbar musculature, most consistent with severe inflammation.

Final diagnosis: Paralumbar abscessation, cellulitis/myositis, and spondylitis. Myelitis of the lumbar spinal cord.

CASE 3.54

1 What are your radiographic findings? There is abnormal ossification and fragmentation of the glenoid cavity of the scapula and a misshapen humeral head. The lumbar vertebrae are shortened with nonossification of the vertebral endplates.
2 What is your radiographic diagnosis? Diffuse skeletal disease principally characterized by epiphyseal dysplasia. A primary differential diagnosis is mucopolysaccharidosis.

Comment: Mucopolysaccharidosis is a recessive inherited disease of lysomal storage disease in dogs and cats. This results in a metabolic deficit of glycosaminoglycans, important for normal joint maturation and maintenance.

CASE 3.55

1 What are your radiographic findings? Left: moderate osteophyte formation is present along the dorsodistal aspect of the radius, dorsodistal aspect of the radiointermediate carpal bone, and dorsal aspect of the distal row of carpal bones. Two osseous bodies are present in the dorsal aspect of the radiocarpal joint, one round and smoothly marginated and the other more linear in shape, smaller and faintly mineralized. These osseous bodies are consistent with synovial osteochondromatosis. Moderate enthesophyte formation is present along the distal aspect of the accessory carpal bone. Moderate irregularly marginated new bone production is present along the lateral and medial aspects of the diaphysis of the first phalanx of the 3rd and 4th digits. Mild to moderate periarticular osteophyte formation is present along the proximal interphalangeal joints of the 2nd, 3rd, and 4th digits and along the metacarpophalangeal joints of the 2nd to 5th digits.

Right: moderate osteophyte formation is present along the dorsodistal aspect of the radius, dorsodistal aspect of the radiointermediate carpal bone, and dorsal aspect of the distal row of carpal bones. Moderate enthesophyte formation is present along the distal aspect of the accessory carpal bone. A moderate amount of irregularly marginated new bone production is present along the lateral and medial aspects of the diaphysis of the first phalanx of the 3rd, 4th, and 5th digits. Moderate periarticular osteophyte formation is also present along the proximal interphalangeal joints of the 3rd to 5th digits and the metacarpophalangeal joint of the 5th digit.

2 **What is your radiographic diagnosis?** Moderate bilateral carpal osteoarthritis; mild to moderate bilateral metacarpophalangeal and proximal interphalangeal osteoarthritis.

Comment: Carpal osteoarthritis is a common finding in middle aged to older dogs. The classic radiographic signs of osteoarthritis include the following: effusion/synovial proliferation, osteophyte/enthesophyte formation, joint space narrowing, subchondral sclerosis, intra-articular soft tissue mineralization, and subchondral cyst formation. Osteophytes are small, periarticular bony projections. Enthesophytes are small, bony projections at the site of soft tissue attachments, such as ligaments, tendons, or a joint capsule. As an additional note, joint space narrowing can be difficult to evaluate in small animal patients as they are not typically nonweight-bearing during the examination and positioning can create an artifactual widening/narrowing of the joint.

CASE 3.56

1 **What are your radiographic findings?** Smoothly marginated bridging osseous callus is present circumferentially along the proximal diaphysis of the tibia, in the region of the previous fracture. The fracture margins are poorly defined. There is mild medial angulation of the tibial diaphysis at the level of the fracture. The distal tibia, tarsal bones, and proximal metatarsal bones have a marked reduction in

mineral opacity, thinning of the cortices, and coarse trabeculation, consistent with disuse osteopenia.

2 What is your radiographic diagnosis? Healed left tibial diaphyseal fracture; marked disuse osteopenia.

Comment: Osteopenia occurs secondary to many conditions, including hyperparathyroidism, disuse, nutritional disorders, neoplasia, or developmental disorders (i.e. osteogenesis imperfecta). Radiographic features of osteopenia include an overall decrease in bone opacity, thinning of the cortices, a coarse trabcular pattern, and possible pathologic fractures.

Radiographs of the normal right tibia of this dog are shown for comparison (**Figs. 3.56c, d**).

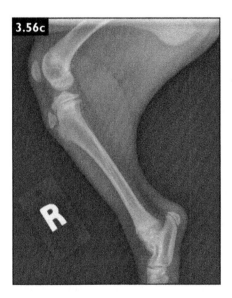 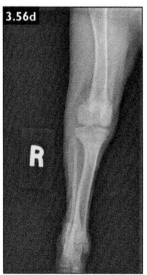

CASE 3.57

1 What are your radiographic findings? There is bridging, flowing bone along the dorsal cervical spine and ventrally along the thoracic spine. Severe periarticular bone accumulation of one shoulder and one elbow is present.

2 What is your radiographic diagnosis? Diffuse, severe metabolic bone disease. Given the history of a lifelong liver diet, a diagnosis of hypervitaminosis A can be made.

Final diagnosis: Hypervitaminosis A.

CASE 3.58

1 What are your radiographic findings? An oblique fracture is present through the body of the right mandible, extending caudal to the last mandibular molar. This fracture is medially and ventrally displaced. No additional fractures are identified. The temporomandibular joints are within normal limits.

2 What is your radiographic diagnosis? Oblique right mandibular fracture.

Comment: Fractures of the skull, including the mandible, are commonly the result of trauma. Oblique views are helpful in determining the extent and orientation of the fractures. If radiographs are not conclusive, a computed tomography examination of the skull may be needed prior to surgical repair of the fracture.

CASE 3.59

1 What are your radiographic findings? A large, well-mineralized, round mass is present along the left dorsolateral aspect of the caudal C1 and cranial C2 vertebrae. Osteolysis of the craniolateral aspect of the C2 vertebral body and spinous process is evident. There is also osteolysis of the left transverse process and body of C1. The C1-2 articulation is widened along the left lateral aspect. A small amount of irregularly marginated osseous proliferation is present along the caudal aspect of the occipital bone of the skull. Also of note, on the lateral view, multiple soft tissue to osseous nodules are present in the cranial pulmonary parenchyma.

2 What is your radiographic diagnosis? Locally invasive, osteolytic mass of the cranial cervical spine (C1-2) most consistent with neoplasia; multiple pulmonary nodules, most consistent with metastatic disease.

3 Are additional radiographs needed? Radiographs of the thorax could be performed to determine the extent of metastasis.

Comment: Axial osteosarcoma has been reported in the mandible, maxilla, cranium, spine, ribs, nasal cavity, sternum, and pelvis. Axial osteosarcoma is not as common as appendicular osteosarcoma and may be more difficult to treat, as surgical removal is often more challenging. Magnetic resonance imaging or computed tomography could be used to determine the severity of compression of adjacent tissues, such as the brain and spinal cord, and invasion into surrounding tissues.

    Final diagnosis: Osteosarcoma of the cervical spine with metastasis.

CASE 3.60

1 What are your radiographic findings? Smoothly marginated mineral opacity is present within the intervertebral disk space of C5-6. Very small, pinpoint foci of mineral opacity are also present in the intervertebral disk space of C4-5.

No additional abnormalities of the cervical spine are identified. The esophageal stethoscope and endotracheal tube are present as the patient is under general anesthesia.

2 What is your radiographic diagnosis? Mineralized C4-5 and C5-6 intervertebral disks.

Comment: Mineralization of the intervertebral disk is a finding associated with degeneration of the disk and commonly seen in chondrodystrophic breeds, such as the Dachshund. However, disk mineralization does not always correlate with the site of intervertebral disk protrusion/herniation/extrusion into the vertebral canal. The typical pattern of mineralization is to start centrally within the nucleus pulposus and continue peripherally.

Normally on T2-weighted magnetic resonance images, the intervertebral disks are hydrated and hyperintense. On the T2 sagittal image from this dog (**Fig. 3.60c**), the intervertebral disks of C5-6 and C6-7 are hypointense, which indicates dessication and possible mineralization. Also note that the disks are bulging dorsally into the ventral aspect of the vertebral canal, causing spinal cord compression.

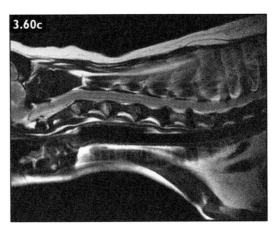

3.60c

Index

Note: References are to case numbers.

Index

Printed and bound by CPI Group (UK) Ltd, Croydon, CR0 4YY

23/10/2024

. 01777696-0003